Nourishing

YOUR BODY & SOUL

JULIE HEFNER

Nourishing

YOUR BODY & SOUL

DEDICATION

To my kids, Brenden, Kate, and Claire. You are all amazing humans, and I love you more than anything. Thank you for your unconditional love and support while I was going back to school. I will always cherish the times we sat at our dining table doing homework together.

Being your mom has been one of the greatest gifts in my life. I am so proud of the incredible people you have become. You all have incredible gifts that God has blessed you with. Don't be afraid to share them. The world needs those gifts. I am so honored and proud to be your mom, and I love you from the bottom of my heart.

To my partner and best friend, Bryan. Thank you for your continued love and support. You have supported me from day one and made me feel like I could accomplish anything in life. You are my rock.

To my mom, Sylvia. You always worked so hard to provide healthy meals for us kids while we were growing up, in spite of not having a lot of money. Even while working two jobs, you found the time to cook healthy meals. This has always been your way of showing love, and I love you for this. Thank you for always being there for me.

To my stepdad, Dave. Thank you for raising me like I was your own daughter. You stepped up in a time in life when I needed it and provided me with unconditional love, guidance, support, and structure. I will always be grateful for this.

To my beautiful sister Kim. Thank you for always being there for me with your daily support and encouragement.

We all have that one person in life that is our biggest cheerleader. For me, that person was my Aunt Mary. You have always believed in me and saw something in me before I even realized it was there. You are loving, supportive, and always speaking my love language, words of affirmation. Thank you, Aunt Mary.

CONTENTS

PART FIVE: ADDITIONAL RESOURCES

A NOTE FROM THE AUTHOR

First, I want to thank you for buying this book. Should you choose to, you are about to change your life. *Or* you will make at least a few changes that will greatly benefit your life.

All around the world, people spend millions of dollars on life-changing books that end up sitting on their shelves forever. What gives? Why do we buy a book and then not read it? Do we get too busy? No, it's because, even though we have the intention to change, by the time we actually read the book, our motivation has faded.

But not this time.

Throughout this book, I'm going to teach you ways to navigate when motivation fades or boredom sets in. I'm happy that you're looking for an opportunity to improve at least one area of your life, and that you chose me!

Second, I wrote this book on health because I want to share my journey with you. I want women to know that they are not alone in striving for their healthiest body. There are women just like you and me who are feeling the same frustration, uncertainty, and overwhelming sensations! You are not alone, and this book will show you that.

I, too, have struggled with creating healthy habits, releasing old ones, battling my inner thoughts, and trying to change. I've come out the other side, and I know that you can too.

After reading this book, my hope is that you will have at least three takeaways from the transformative content that I'm about to share with you. As you're reading, feel free to write in this book, and fill out all the blank spots that I'm providing you.

If you're one of those people who likes to keep your books and workbooks pristine, I'm the same! But you know what? Sometimes we need to make it messy to actually do the work, so I encourage you to write in this book. Make it your companion! Take it everywhere if you have to. Leave it out on the kitchen counter. Do whatever you have to to make yourself successful. If you don't want to write in it, then I strongly recommend writing in a separate notebook. In fact, grab one right now so you can take a few notes.

This is going to be worth it.

Nourishing

YOUR BODY & SOUL

THE POWER OF NOURISHING YOURSELF

I'm the youngest of three kids, but also the strongest. I needed to be. As a kid, I was pretty adventurous and tough, but had a sensitive and warm side. Like most of my clients, I had battles to fight from the very beginning.

When I was five years old, my parents split up. My dad wasn't home often. Eventually, my mom realized that he was having an affair, prompting their divorce. He moved an hour away, so I saw him even less. The divorce left me feeling like I was different than everyone else, like I was incomplete.

After that, we didn't have a lot of money. My mom worked two jobs until she met my stepdad, Dave, who ended up raising me because I didn't have much contact with my real dad. We left my childhood home to move in with Dave, in a new community for all of us. At first, the change seemed scary and different.

Moving from the city to the country completely changed my environment. It forced me to learn more about myself. Eventually, the new move made my life more adventurous. I made friends quickly and enjoyed living in the country.

My life became a flow of constant change. I've had my share of past difficulties, but I acclimated and overcame. Change, difficult circumstances, and breaking through unhealthy habits is probably common in your life, too. That's a great thing! Because when you stop and look back, those little moments of pain or trauma help make us who we are.

I know you can work through it too.

Becoming Stronger

No one in my family had graduated high school or college, and I was determined to be the first. The day after graduating from high school, I moved to the beach to attend a local junior college and fulfill my dream. Eventually, I managed a clothing store while attending day and night classes. One day, my stepdad called.

"Julie," he said. "There's a great opportunity to become an outside sales representative at a local title company. I really think you should take it."

The current sales representative was going on maternity leave, so it was going to be a temporary position. (Or so I thought.) The money was better, and the work excited me. I got the job and started to work. That "temporary job" turned into two years, until I finally transferred to another company closer to home. My college education temporarily halted in the face of greater financial stability and being closer to home. Getting my own apartment, making money, setting goals, and being with my girlfriends sidetracked my motivation for a college degree.

At the time, my body was healthy, thin, and I did a little modeling as well. All these positive things helped me build up my confidence and self-worth. Life was good! I had control of my life and couldn't wait to see what came next.

When I met a nice-looking guy while out with my friends at twenty-one years old, it only seemed to get better.

Jack and I first met in passing, and I didn't think much of him. Later, he approached me with a quick smile and a funny wit and definitely caught my attention.

The next day, he called my company. They paged me (yes, that totally dates this story!), and sent me his number to call him back. He was *working* for more time with me! I felt incredibly special. This time, he asked me out. I agreed. During our first date, he made me laugh so hard I spit out some of my salad.

More dates followed. Jack opened my door and made me laugh. He was a polite gentleman who made me feel respected, cared for, and protected.

One day while eating at a restaurant, Jack turned to me and said, "You eat a lot for a girl. I've never seen anything like it."

I set my fork down, unsure of what to say. The subject changed, and I didn't think much more of it. Later, when I pulled on a pair of his old Levi's that he let me wear, they stayed on without the belt I normally used. Without giving it much thought, I left them on.

While out shopping together, I passed a scale. "Look!" I said, pointing. "I want to see what it says."

The numbers 138 popped onto the screen. My eyes widened. *How did that happen?* I thought. When we started dating, I had been 121. His jaw dropped.

"Whoa," he said. "That's how much my mom weighs!"

Frustration filled me. His mom was a lot bigger than me, so it didn't seem right that we were the same weight. I brushed his comment off—surely, he didn't mean that. Only later would I learn that had been a lie and a gross exaggeration. Because we went out to dinner all the time (and ordered dessert as a rule), the calories had clearly started to add up.

As we walked through the store, a feeling of confusion filled me. Something had to be done, but what? How was I supposed to lose weight? I'd never had to do it before, and I had no clue what to do.

I looked for weight loss clinics in my neighborhood. When I found one, I went and signed up immediately. Every week I came home with shelf-stable, tiny meals wrapped in plastic that made it so I didn't have to think about food. (Or chemicals, additives, or learning anything about the process of being healthier.) The little plates would stack up in the kitchen as I collected them, dutifully obeying what they told me to do, but not really making any other sort of change.

Thanks to sticking with something and having someone to check in with each week, I lost some weight. The power of meeting with the staff in the weight loss clinic surprised me—having them to talk about this process made a difference! Still, I didn't *feel* good. Internally, I felt no happier. My body wasn't truly nourished, but I hadn't realized that yet.

Big surprise, but that kind of an approach to health didn't help—certainly not for the long-term. I didn't learn any skills when someone gave me food to eat. I walked away from the weight loss clinic thinking I shouldn't eat dessert or appetizers, and having a basic idea of better portion sizes. In the end, I was less educated and less healthy than before.

Jack and I continued dating for five years before we married. Warning signs started to pop up everywhere, but instead of looking into them, I accepted them as part of him. As an extrovert, he wanted to go out all the time. Being in the home drained his energy. As an introvert, I sometimes struggled with the constant social demand. We traveled all the time, went out to really nice dinners, and spent time with friends, but we didn't have a lot of time at home together. We were always on the go, having fun. At the end of the day, though, we ended up with little connection between us.

My dream of graduating college faded into the background as life progressed with Jack. I'd think about it, but push it away. College could come later. And who needed it, anyway? Eventually, we spoke about having a family.

Thanks to a removed ovary with an enlarged cyst, I wasn't confident that I could get pregnant. Stress over whether I could have a child led me back to food. My lack of education on how to truly nourish myself meant I didn't know *how* to eat, *what* to eat, or *when* to eat it. Nutrients or quality food weren't part of the plan. I ended up gaining fifteen pounds trying to conceive, and then I gained forty pounds while pregnant with my first. When I delivered our son, my weight had crept up to 185.

I'm eating for two, I remember thinking as I opened the refrigerator and reached inside. *I can eat two breakfasts or lunches!*

Despite gaining over fifty pounds, my little guy was born at a whopping 6 pounds, 6 ounces. His small size came as a total shock. What the heck! Didn't he take up more of the weight I had gained? Total mom guilt right there.

Not only that, but my stomach had extra fat and skin that hadn't been there before, and I had major stretch marks on my thighs and stomach. *Goodbye body,* I thought with a sinking, heavy feeling in my chest. *Will I ever feel like myself again?*

Deciding that it took nine months for my body to change to this shape and size, I figured I'd have to give myself nine months to take it back off. Starting when my son was six weeks old, I walked with him each day for thirty minutes. Eventually, I increased that time to sixty minutes. I took my measurements and weighed in on my scale. The weight started to come off without intense exercise or pre-packaged meals! I felt pretty good about myself again.

My increased confidence led me back to my initial goal of graduating from college. I signed up for a writing class at our local junior college, ecstatic to have a starting point again. This initial foray back into the educational world left me feeling empowered and ecstatic.

Until I told Jack.

I remember he said to me, "How could you do this to our family? You're going to be away from our son at your class. How selfish can you be?"

That sinking feeling hit my stomach again. Coming from a divorced family meant I never wanted to get divorced, so any hint of trouble left me concerned. My goal was to be the best wife to my husband and mother to my kids. Could I do that while pursuing what I wanted? Despite Jack's objection, I kept to the class. About six weeks into it, I started feeling nauseated.

Surprise, surprise . . . I was pregnant again!

This was the best surprise of my life. Thanks to sickness and the guilty feeling of doing something wrong by being in school as a young mother, I dropped out. Still, questions plagued me.

Was I selfish?

Did I do the wrong thing?

That sounded silly because I was only away three hours all week, and my mom babysat my son, but I questioned whether it *was* the right thing for our family. The question mulled in the back of my mind as I progressed through the pregnancy and gave birth to my daughter.

For a long time, the dichotomy between what I wanted to do and what sounded like the right thing created confusion in my heart. Add stress, a second child, and a turbulent marriage, and my body caught every cold and flu I happened on. I missed being active on family vacations and events because I was always sick.

Time passed. My college dream seemed like a distant memory while I cared for our two children. The marriage continued to spiral down. Trying to be perfect for him and the kids left me feeling numb and exhausted every night. Jack seemed to criticize everything I did or said. He left all the time after work, leaving me alone with the kids and the household. I never felt like I was enough.

After delivering my third child, my stomach had some flabby skin. One night, a look of revulsion crossed Jack's face when he saw me shirtless. I'll never forget when he said, "Your stomach grosses me out." I turned away, horrified, humiliated, and hurt.

Thankfully, while in a women's Bible study group with ten other women, I shared some of the things that were happening at home.

"That," one of them said with a look of concern, "isn't normal."

"Or healthy," chimed in another. "You deserve to be treated better!"

I had no idea how bad it had gotten until they helped me see the stress and toll my marriage had on me. Once again, the power of other people helped me. Of course, marriage is hard no matter how well matched you are. Ups and downs are to be expected, but our relationship was clearly out of the norm. I felt totally lost, helpless, and alone.

My health continued to take a nosedive into a bloated abdomen, exhaustion, and being run down at the end of the day. By then, I was in my thirties, with three children and no self-esteem. Physical exhaustion plagued me on a daily basis. In a last-ditch effort to take care of myself, I hired a personal trainer. He insisted that I eat whole grain products instead of white products. Instead of white rice, I swapped for brown. Instead of white bread, I chose multigrain. He was on the right track, but missed the mark for *my* body. Despite these changes, I still felt the same way, but now even worse. At this point, I was at the end of my rope.

With the worsening of my gastrointestinal issues, I decided to talk to my doctor and get some allergy testing done.

Eventually, the tests revealed something I never expected—I had allergies to whole grains, eggs, red meat, chocolate, dairy, and soy. Being sick a lot as a kid made so much sense now; I had allergies to foods that I'd been consuming my entire life!

"Allergies?" I said to the doctor. "To *all* of those things?"

I'd never had any rashes or major problems that, to me, indicated allergies. Only quite a bit later, did I eventually see the correlation between my avoiding those foods and not getting sick. Or feeling exhausted. Or having energy to complete my day. My body needed the right kinds of nutrients, not pre-packaged meals or hurried lunches in between taking care of kids. I just didn't see it at the time.

That's when I realized that I needed more than health. I needed to *nourish* myself. This wasn't just about losing weight or looking the best or having a perfect body for my husband.

My goal was for me, and my family, to be healthy.

After that fateful doctor's visit, I switched my eating habits to avoid those specific foods. The value in healing symptoms naturally, instead of through medications, slowly dawned on me. I started shopping at our local health food store and reading labels. As a result of being nourished, my body began the process of healing.

Time passed. I felt better. More like, well . . . *me*. Instead of feeling insecure, lacking confidence, and uncertain, I became empowered. Eating the right foods and taking care of my soul through self-care helped me feel good about myself. Not only did I feel good in my body, but I felt empowered in a marriage where I felt helpless and trodden down constantly. In fact, it seemed like I was nourishing my soul when I took care of my body.

From there, my life started to change.

My body became stronger—both mentally as well as physically. The old way of doing things in our marriage wasn't working for me anymore. I wanted someone that was home with me and the kids. I wanted a partner that was supportive, who didn't make me feel like I was being torn down all the time. My newfound confidence gave me the courage to speak up to my husband.

I made a list of how I wanted to be treated and what wasn't acceptable to me anymore. Then I handed it to Jack and said, "Here it is. If you want to be married, these are my terms."

Several counselors guided us over the next five years, but eventually, we realized that we both wanted different things. It just wasn't going to work. The marriage had ended, trailing into a devastating, crushing, stressful, and long divorce process.

Nourishing Habits

After the divorce, I wasn't sure I could ever be enough.

Could I really start working again, get married a second time, or raise our kids to be happy despite coming from a divorced home? Had I failed? Would I be happy again on my own? Was this the right path? Uncertainties and questions plagued me, but I knew I couldn't stay in that place. I had to do *something*.

In order to give myself the best chance to succeed, I decided to put a few things into place that would ensure my success.

For one, I made the decision to only drink alcohol rarely because I noticed that it messed with my emotions. The day after having alcohol, I'd feel depressed, and my sleep would be off. Cutting that out helped me sleep better, stay more emotionally stable for my kids, and not be so anxious. Making the decision beforehand seemed like it protected me from the effects and made it easier to say *no* to my friends.

Interesting, I thought. I paid attention to the improved way I felt and kept going.

After a while, I realized that I needed to supplement my body with vitamin D3 because I don't produce it from the sun like most people. I started taking a quality supplement to make sure occasional anxiety and depression stayed low. Within days of beginning vitamin D supplementation, I felt a shift in my moods.

Also interesting, I thought. With those two habits firmly in place, I continued on my path, moving to the next thing that helped me cope with my new world better.

Exercise, sleep, vitamins, nourishing food, and empowerment books became part of my normal life. I made sure all these things slipped into place one at a time. *All these habits,* I realized as I looked at my slowly improving life situation, *are nourishing my body and soul.* They were there in the moments I needed them. They protected me. These habits gave me excellent health—which is the greatest freedom of all.

At the time, a deep love for nutrition had started to grow within me. Finally, I felt myself come full circle again: I decided to go back to school for a degree in nutrition. Instead of working, I attended school just like my kids. We even did homework together! My kids were so proud of how strong their mom was. We shared grades, discussed schoolwork, and bought supplies together, making learning more interesting for all of us.

Eventually, I did what I set out to do. I graduated with an Associates of Science degree and a Nutrition Education certificate, making me a certified nutritionist and the first person in my family to graduate from college.

In 2013, I found an office space in Newport Beach, California and founded *Nourish Nutrition and Health.* My goal was to provide education, support, and resources for women like me who needed nourishment and empowerment, not shelf-stable food and shaming.

While working with other women, hearing their stories, and seeing all their struggles with food, themselves, and their habits, I realized the full power of truly nourishing ourselves. Not only did I feel like myself again, but I'd empowered myself through good food to make positive lifestyle changes. Having a community again gave me even greater strength, and I finally thrived while doing what I loved. I had found my passion!

The benefits of nourishing myself extended beyond me. When my kids had issues come up, or they became sick, I would immediately go to food first to help heal them. My clients began to transform their bodies, reach their goals, and shed aliments they had struggled with for years. With education, support, and accountability, my clients had huge successes.

They inspired me! I want that for you, too.

After struggling for years, mentally and physically, the solution ended up coming through my overall health, not just weight loss. Nourishing your body and soul was a key that unlocked happiness and clarity in *all* other aspects of my life. When I turned my focus to nourishment, I became a better person, a better mother, and more . . . I actually began to love myself again. Because of that, I found love again. I met a great guy that loves me unconditionally, and is supportive and kind.

We need to take good health beyond the scale and make sure we're caring for our soul. To address only one facet of your health isn't enough! We need to make sure our bodies and souls get equal attention.

That's where *Nourishing Your Body and Soul* can change your life.

You Are Enough

Life is funny sometimes. We tend to experience the same ups and downs, often in what feels like a cycle.

After years of speaking with clients, I've learned that everything negative that we go through leaves a little mark or tear on our heart and soul. Kind of like a computer hard drive getting worn down, becoming slower and slower until we begin to reach for food or drink to solve our problems. It gives us a little shot of happiness. We rely on it. Then we reach for food to help us sleep. Then help us get out of bed. At some point, we think we can't manage without it.

It's a broken system from the beginning. I've also come to appreciate that having a broken system isn't necessarily a bad thing . . . as long as we use it as feedback. More on that coming soon.

Along the path of my life, I've dealt with many things. My parents' divorce, loved ones tearing me down, my brother dying from issues related to addiction, family trauma, heartache, mistrust, betrayal, loss of a job, discarded dreams, raising three children (although this is also the greatest joy in my life), a struggling marriage, and finally my own heartbreaking divorce. As a Christian woman, I struggled with all the pain. Eventually, I came to terms with it through my relationship with God.

What I learned was that all these experiences forced me to a decision point: I could let the struggle take me down, or I would find a way for it to make me stronger. I could be pushed down by my problems or pulled up toward greatness. Thanks to my struggles, I know I am incredibly strong, and I am a fighter.

You are too.

Not sharing what I've learned along the way would be selfish! That's why this book is coming now. Women need to know how extraordinary they are and how to set themselves up for long-term success. (Without blanket advice and prepackaged meals!)

Through this book, I want to teach you to love yourself no matter what weight you are. To look at food as nutrients that can fuel your body and heal your symptoms, instead of using them as an emotional crutch. I want you to embrace your imperfections, stretch marks, saggy stomach, and whatever else you think makes you not good enough. Chances are, what you've been through is a lot!

And you are enough.

I don't think we hear that—or say it to ourselves—enough.

In fact, here are a few things I want you to start saying to yourself right now:

- I am going to start today.
- Today, I'm going to focus on getting healthy.

- I am going to make better health my lifestyle.
- Getting to the best version of me is a process.
- I will not beat myself up along the way.
- There is no failure, only feedback.

What You Can Expect

In *Nourishing Your Body and Soul,* we focus on being healthy in your body and your soul. (Doesn't that sound so much better than saying, "I'm on a diet"?) We can't take the soul out of this work, or else our body won't really thrive!

This book will teach you how to establish safety within your own habits and how to take care of yourself. I mean *truly* take care of yourself. I don't just mean losing weight or squeezing in a manicure every six months as an act of self-care. With greater overall health comes more abiding happiness, which means you can fulfill your life purpose with greater intention. This isn't just about you. Think of all the people you can impact.

Through this book, I want to empower you to make a change. Just one change can make our world a happier, better place. It will only ripple out from there. Together, let's rise up and work on our body and soul so we become radiant. Because when we are radiant, we can help lift others up by giving back.

Nourishing Your Body and Soul is a stepping-stone. This method isn't a prescription—I can't tell you exactly what to do, what to eat, when to eat it, and expect you to have long-term success. Everyone is different. The term "healthy" is defined by the individual, not a saran-wrapped diet.

That's why my goal is to make recommendations that help you find *your* solution, not the solution of the masses or the latest fad. Customizing your plan to your body is the best approach to being and staying healthy. No more quick fixes. Together, we can get to the root of the problem so you feel your best, prevent future disease, and positively impact the world.

Having me as your guide creates an instant community. You're not alone, and the stories of other women that I've worked with will help you see that.

I've structured the book so it's easy to skip around to the part you want—even though I encourage you to start at the beginning and work forward. If you want to speed right ahead to the science, just turn to Part Two. If you want to initiate your plan immediately, go to Part Four. You'll find resources to help you put it all together in Part Five.

Let's nourish your body with nutrients for a long and healthy life. Allow yourself to succeed this time. With the right support, guidance, time, and grace, you can reach your goals. I've seen it happen. Not only in my own life but working with hundreds of women from different lifestyles and needs.

First, you must believe that you will succeed!

This *magic pill* is nothing more than setting yourself up for success with nourishing habits. If you allow yourself to be successful, you become unstoppable. When you feel good about yourself, you do good things. You take decisive action. You care for yourself and your family better. You experience a level of life you didn't have before.

That is the power of nourishing yourself.

PART ONE

THE
Solution
TO GOOD
HEALTH

CHAPTER 1

WHAT'S YOUR WHY?

Women who come to me are of all ages and sizes. Almost all of them have one thing in common: they need help getting to their healthiest body.

They've tried before, but it's never worked. Or it's worked . . . but they've gained the weight back and then some. Diets and eating plans and online gurus and quick-weight-loss promises abound all over TV, radio, and the internet. Most of my clients have tried most (or all) of those impersonal gimmicks. They're based on a broad group, not on the individual. Good health is not one-size-fits-all.

How can you focus on an individual person with all their idiosyncrasies when you give a basic plan? If I gave you an eating plan, it might not work. I don't know all *your* details to even make the right plan. Then you'd declare yourself a failure, say you *just can't lose weight*, and possibly turn back to unhealthy foods to cope. What if your hormones or your habits were the problem, but you didn't see that? An eating plan would be a band-aid—a temporary surface-level solution that wouldn't bring the desired results.

That's why I work one-on-one to help people figure out *their* best path. I firmly believe that when you have the knowledge, you will make the right decisions. (Most of the time!) The first part of that is figuring out why you're doing this.

Why did you pick up this book? Why are you seeking something better? Beneath all of our surface-level desires lurks something infinitely more valuable to us. Perhaps we're trying to ease pain from a loss, or be around for our grandchildren, or have more energy to change the world through our careers.

When my health hit an all-time low after my third child, it forced me to ask hard questions like *why do I want to be healthier?*

The answer, although it required time to figure out, was pretty simple:

1. I didn't want to feel sick and tired anymore.
2. I wanted to look my best.
3. I wanted energy to play with my kids.

Ultimately, my *why* is to live a long and healthy life so I can have fun with my kids and, someday, my grandkids. I don't want to miss a second of it! I want to be present, healthy, and a solid example for those I love.

What started as a diet thing eventually turned out to be a huge eye-opener into my health. Consider it a journey of self-discovery. At the time, I thought it was just about my body, but it became so much more. I felt strong and empowered. I felt alive. My life had purpose. Better nutrients going into my body brought more optimal health.

Right now, I want to ask you something you may not have been asked before: **Why are you doing this?**

Why did you pick up this book? Why do you want to be healthier? Why make changes? Why do you want to try this version of getting healthy? Are you hoping to have a bikini body? Do you want greater longevity? Better skin? Are you tired of struggling or being on a diet all the time? Have you wondered if there was a better way?

What is it you truly want? Do you want joy, love, confidence, peace, romance, to be respected, to be adored? Have you had that in the past and lost it . . . or maybe never had it at all?

Is it to meet a quality partner, and you need confidence? Or is it to get that dream job or start your own business? Do you want to travel, and you're broke?

That can all change!

Figuring out your why is key to your own success, and it has to be the first thing you do before you dive into the rest of this book. Take a moment to sit down and write any of your reasons for wanting better health.

Here are a few responses that I often see from my clients:

1. Lose weight.

2. Sleep better.

3. Have healthier skin.

4. Heal my digestive tract.

5. Increase my confidence.

6. Improve my fitness.

7. Fix my nutrition.

8. Better health.

9. More energy.

10. Prevent disease.

Decide your motivation now so you can remember it in your darkest moments. Write it on your hand, your wall, your mirror. Say it out loud every morning. The stronger your motivation, the stronger your will.

You can have your why. You can have everything you want. Your own journey of self-discovery and soul-nourishment starts in your mind, not your body. Your body is just a result of work that the mind achieved.

Know Yourself

Can you be successful if you don't know yourself? It's a question I ask all the time—and I see the answer in every client that I work with. The short answer is *no*. If you don't know yourself, you will have a harder time being successful.

Nourishing yourself is all about getting to *know* yourself. How can you nourish your soul if you don't know what fills you up? How can you nourish your body when you don't know what you need?

Figuring out your *why* was the best first step . . . but I want to push you a little further. The following exercise may not feel comfortable, but that's what I want from you. Get uncomfortable. Go to those places you don't normally go in your mind so you can discover yourself. This is exactly what makes my method different than everyone else.

Figuring out your why goes beyond why you're seeking a healthier life. It should dive right into everything *behind* your why.

Now, grab a new sheet of paper, and write down your answers to these questions:

1. What is it that I really want?

   ----

2. How do I want to feel and look?

   ----

3. What is getting in my way?

   ----

4. What are my beliefs around reaching my goals?

5. Have I tried before, and it hasn't worked, so I think it won't this time?

6. What are the things that sabotage me from getting what I want?

7. Why am I doing things I know aren't good for me?

8. Do I kick ass in other areas of life, but can't ever seem to achieve this one specific thing?

9. Do I blame my lack of success on my body or family genetics?

10. Do I eat or drink to feel better?

11. What am I hiding from?

12. Can I really *see* my goal? (For example, if you want radiant skin, can you imagine looking in the mirror and finding it? Or waking up in the morning feeling rested—not exhausted?)

Once you finish answering those questions, sit back, and look at your responses for a minute. Allow yourself to think through them and *feel* the emotions they bring. Has anything surprised you? If you can't picture it, why? Is there something standing in your way?

Let's look at Lori, an example that represents a lot of the clients I work with.

"Julie," Lori told me when we first started meeting. "At the end of the day, I just want to have a glass of wine. It helps me wind down after dealing with work, the kids, and my messy house all day long."

"But why do you *have to* have the wine?" I asked, challenging her dependence. "Could you survive without it?"

A puzzled expression came to her face. "I guess. I could *survive*, yes."

"Wine affects your sleep. It may not seem like it, but you won't sleep as well after drinking wine."

"But how else will I wind down?" she asked. "My glass of wine gives me something to look forward to so I can just get through the day. It relaxes me."

What Lori didn't realize is that *just getting through the day* isn't normal. We shouldn't have to white-knuckle our way through our lives! Sometimes we don't even realize that that's exactly what we're doing.

As women, we're always serving the other people in our lives. Most of the time, we're catering to or serving others instead of ourselves. We purchase the groceries, cook, and meal plan. We work, take care of kiddos, check on everyone, and clean the house. By the end of the day, it's no wonder we think we need a drink to calm down!

There's a belief among my clients who depend on something at the end of the day (whether it's wine, chocolate, sugar, or chips) that they *have* to have it. But they don't. In fact, they've believed it for so long, and it's so ingrained in our culture, that they think this is normal.

It's not! It's not *normal* to want wine every single night. Those are the kind of beliefs I want you to find through making this list. Then we're going to uproot them so you can move past them; otherwise, your success may be short-lived.

My client, Susan, came into my office for her first appointment. She sat down, looked me in the eye, and said, "I drink wine every night. It's how I relax after work. So is ice cream. I drink wine, eat ice cream, and have a treat at work sometimes. It's like I can't stop eating sugar."

After one week of instilling more nourishing habits, she cut way back on wine and sugar. After a while, she hit a plateau. Her progress toward a healthier life had stalled so soon after starting. "The only thing left to do is completely cut out the wine," I said to Susan. "Are you willing to try it?"

By this time, she was ready. She completely gave up wine and sugar for six months. One day she came in, slammed her hand on my desk, and said, "I no longer have a relationship with sugar! I don't crave it at all. Not even at a dessert table at a wedding."

That is far more normal. In fact, Susan had gained so much confidence she was planning to fly to Hawaii for the first time alone. My program had given her an accurate sense of normal, as well as some confidence. She ended up losing a total of thirty-five pounds and completely stopped drinking wine, which improved her sleep and stopped her hot flashes.

To take yourself to the next level, I want you to question everything you think is normal. Drinking wine at night. Having a cup of coffee in the morning. Craving chocolate or something sweet at the end of every meal. Feeling too tired to sleep at night. Needing a nap at 2:00 p.m. Drinking a cup of coffee or soda every day. Maybe it's normal for you—but it's actually a sign from our body that something isn't working.

Maybe you think you're not stressed, but is that *really* true? Is it normal to binge eat a box of cookies? To sleep until ten in the morning and still be tired? The more you question, the deeper the layers you're likely to find. It may be difficult, but I promise it will be worth it.

Question, question, question.

We have to be our own advocate if we want to reach our healthiest bodies, and figuring out why you're doing this is the first step. It will keep you motivated through the hard times, so be ready to return to your why when you need the reminder. Feel free to list any thoughts below that have cropped up as you read.

_____

_____

_____

_____

There Is No Failure, Only Feedback

If, during the course of nourishing your body and soul, you stumble or think you've failed, then great job!

Maybe you didn't expect to hear that. You probably won't hear anyone else saying this, but I need you to fail at least once when you start on this journey to better health. It's hard to find that permission in the nutrition world, but I'm here to say that, in fact, it's *really good* to fail. One of my favorite sayings is, "There is no failure, only feedback."

The truth is this: we all need to fail. Failing isn't bad.

When doing something new, I expect you to stumble a little bit. We're all human! The sooner you accept it, the better. Failing helps you figure out a plan. I've seen other nutritionists help people lose weight through a really hardcore methodology. They have a plan, a meal calendar, and tell you exactly what they want you to do for a specific amount of time. But then their clients don't know what to do after the program ends. What happens next? Do they have to stay on that plan forever?

Is that sustainable?

They didn't work through the hard stuff of daily decisions when they didn't have the food calendar, repeated failures getting back onto the healthy bandwagon, and the mindset issues that crop up. If I give you a plan that is proven to work, but I don't help you through real-life application, then I'm setting you up to fail.

One of my clients, Leslie, said to me on a call one day, "I feel like I'm constantly in a cycle. I do so good, then something happens, even if it's small, and I drop off the bandwagon. Then I have to climb back on. Sometimes it's easy; sometimes it's not. Sometimes it's fast; sometimes it's slow. Is it normal to cycle like this all the time? I feel like my highs are so high, and then I just start dropping so fast. Does this get easier?"

"Almost every client does this," I said. "They're doing great, just going along, and everything's fine. Their nourishing habits are in place. And then, all of a sudden, something comes up. We have triggers, we have mindset issues, and we have lives. It's not failure. It's just feedback."

With a little more discussion, Leslie realized she hadn't failed. She'd simply found more feedback to make her next step more successful. Not only that, but she learned another way to give herself grace (which is also something else we'll talk about later!)

When I work one-on-one with clients for six to twelve months, I expect them to find a path to their healthiest body. Along that route, I also expect them to fail a few times and then learn from it. They come up with their own meal plan that incorporates food that they like, or they try out different types of exercise. With my guidance, they figure out their trigger foods so they can plan ways to avoid them.

Shame isn't the best motivator long-term, so don't fall into that trap as you move into the nourishing habits we'll practice together. If you're being hard on yourself while initiating new things, then stop. Give yourself some grace. Take a deep breath. Say to yourself, "There is no failure, only feedback."

Failure is only failure when we stop trying to really nourish ourselves.

You're a busy woman with important relationships, a career or business, and dreams to achieve. The world doesn't have time for you to beat yourself up. Getting feedback and learning about yourself makes the lessons really stick. That is sustainable and healthy change we can keep tapping into.

What makes *Nourishing Your Body and Soul* different is that I've built opportunities for feedback (or when you "fall off the bandwagon") into the book. Once you waver, I'll show you how to get back to nourishing yourself. Sometimes, we have to learn to be our own cheerleaders.

> "Our struggles are the short-term steps we must take on our way to long-term success."
> –Simon Sinek

Too Much Information

Before we dive into nourishing habits, let's address the fact that there is *so much information* out there. And, it's almost always conflicting information!

The amount of studies, advice, and programs available is even confusing for me. We read one thing that says spinach is good for us and then one article that it isn't. One study says that coconut oil is a miracle food, but another says it's horribly harmful. What gives? What do you do in such a confusing world with so much information?

Here is what you do: you figure out how your body feels when you try something.

Do you feel good eating that sugary donut? (Not what are you *thinking*, what are you *feeling*!) Check your symptoms. Allow your body to tell you how it feels instead of using your emotions to decide. Normal looks like easy control, not emotions.

You can read one scientific paper, then find it refuted by another. Just when one eating strategy starts to make sense, another one pops up, or studies come out to show that both are wrong. Don't get lost in the chaos, which is all too easy to do.

How do you stay stable?

I tell all my clients to keep a few things in mind if they end up with information overload:

1. If it feels good and is working for you without adverse effects, do that thing. What works for you may not work for someone else.

2. Your body wants homeostasis and support. In working to find your healthiest body, keep that in the back of your mind. Too much exercise, but no rest, is not supportive. Too little exercise and too much rest also aren't supportive. Neither moves us toward homeostasis. Keep your eye on helping the body find homeostasis.

3. The way we should feel is in control, with energy, and no cravings. This is normal. So few people actually live in a place of control that most people don't even know what it feels like. Try to find that feeling every day.

4. Keep in mind your life stage. There are other factors that play into how your body deals with stress, and we'll discuss those. A brand-new college student has different needs than a woman in menopause. If you need more help, don't hesitate to reach out to me at info. nourishyourbody@gmail.com.

5. Test these things for yourself. Tune into your own body. What feels best? What foods don't feel good? What exercise is too straining? We are figuring this out for you, not for anyone else, so don't be afraid to customize and test.

As you read this book, or others, you can find info to support whatever you want. That's why I advocate that the best thing to do is to know yourself. Question the state of your body. Figure out what works for you. Knowing where you are in life and what's going on in your body will set you up for success because *you* are creating *your* blueprint.

You'll know if something is working by the feedback it gives you. Learn your own body. Pay attention to the way you feel and the way your body reacts.

Then take that information and nourish yourself, body and soul.

A quick note: *I am not a doctor and this book is for informational purposes only. Any medical advice you need or want to take should always be discussed with them. My book is intended to educate you with alternatives centered around nourishing practices. Don't wait to see a doctor if you have a problem, but the information I provide in this book are all things you can try in the meantime or rule out with your doctor's guidance.*

CHAPTER 2

NOURISHING HABITS

When you travel down the interstate, you probably don't even pay attention to the guardrails on either side.

They take various forms—whether they're thick, concrete barriers that prevent you from plunging off a dangerous cliff, or metal railings that separate lanes of traffic. Regardless of whether or not you pay attention to them, they're there. They provide safety, and they also give you room to breathe.

I like to think of nourishing habits as guardrails. If you "crash" into an old habit (meaning you're tempted by that luscious slice of chocolate cake or you decide to skip lunch to make it to a last-minute meeting), you're still protected by your habits. We might bump up against the guardrails, but we don't go over them. They're there to protect us.

Nourishing habits are the same thing.

As women, our focus is usually to make money and/or take care of our family, but we also have to take care of ourselves. That's why I help busy women come up with their own nourishing habits. When we protect our health and ourselves, we're really protecting our family, our businesses, and all those we impact.

Here is an example: let's say you purchase a large bag of tortilla chips. Instead of taking the entire bag to the couch and turning on the TV, check the serving size and put that amount in a bowl or baggie. When you're in the habit of awareness and portion control, it protects you from feeling sick or overloading your body with unnecessary foods.

Here are the nourishing habits I advocate for all of my clients. We'll dive further into each of these throughout this book, as well as give you ways to implement them. These aren't comprehensive. There are countless nourishing habits to use, but these are the best ones to start with.

Nourishing Habits for Your Body

1. **Protect your sleep.** If you start the day already tired, you'll fight a losing battle all day long. Not only will you be more likely to eat when you aren't hungry, but not getting enough sleep causes a chain reaction of other hormonal issues.
2. **Drink warm water with lemon every morning.** This helps to detox your body, clean out your liver, and prevent you from starting the day dehydrated.
3. **Ensure you have 8-10 glasses of water per day.** Oftentimes, we turn to food instead of water when we're actually thirsty. (Seems kind of backward, doesn't it?) Without enough water, you don't feel as good, you'll feel more fatigued, and you'll be more likely to seek sugary foods to wake up.
4. **Fast at least twelve hours every night.** Have a twelve-hour fast (or a period of time where you don't eat) at

night. Think 7:00 p.m.-7:00 a.m. As long as you're eating enough calories during the day, cutting off your eating a few hours before bedtime can be beneficial. We'll go deeper into why later.

5. **Eat three macro-balanced meals a day.** I always emphasize protein, fat, and fiber. Look at your plate at every meal. What does it need more of?

6. **Weight loss.** Finding your healthiest weight isn't as easy as looking at a scale, because every body is different. We want you to find the place where you feel great and your health reflects that from the inside out.

7. **Keep your insulin down.** The advice to *eat every two hours* has led many health-seekers astray. When we eat constantly, we cause a rollercoaster for our insulin and energy levels. Instead, consume three balanced meals, while keeping sugar intake low.

Nourishing Habits for Your Soul

1. **Gratitude.** Expressing gratitude is a powerful way to create motivation and move you out of the places of despair we sometimes become stuck in. Focus on all that you do have, not what is missing.

2. **Positive self-talk.** The mean things we say to ourselves would shock many people if we said them out loud. One of the greatest ways to truly nourish ourselves is to pay attention to the narrative in our head—and be far kinder than we are now.

3. **Exercise.** This doesn't have to be strenuous, and you don't have to jump into a rigorous program. Going for a walk, a swim, or finding other ways to move your body can do amazing things for your health. The goal is to get at least 10,000 steps a day. If you are absolutely opposed to exercise, start with window shopping. That's my favorite!

4. **Limit stress.** This may feel like a lot to ask, but it's a crucial step. Many of us create our own stress, or force our bodies to survive on it. Not only does it affect our physical health, but our emotional health as well.

5. **Self-care.** Women are horrible at taking care of themselves! We can't show up in the world, ready to be our best, healthiest selves if we're starving for a little pampering. It's time to give it to ourselves. Self-care is not selfish.

6. **Celebrate your wins.** It's all so easy to focus on the bad things that happen or the failures that seem to pile up. But one easy hack can lead us to a brighter, more successful world: counting all our wins in the day.

7. **Give yourself grace.** The pursuit of perfectionism is rampant and ruining our happiness. Accepting that we're imperfect will feed our soul and set us up for greater success later.

Keep in mind that your nourishing habits are here to create safety in the moments when motivation fails or life crashes into you. That means that as you place these safety zones into your life, there will be change. You have to create these habits before you see them start to work effectively (even though you can see results within a day or two.)

This may not always feel like an easy process. It often takes trial and error as we gain feedback about how your body works. For example, a sweet lady named Sara came to me one day. She was very thin, well dressed, and sent to me by referral from her doctor.

"I'm not at a healthy enough weight," she said. "I need to gain more. The problem could be my blood sugar."

Sara and I created a balanced eating plan that would supply all the nutrients she needed, as well as enough nourishment to provide her with some extra pounds to her frame. Together, we created her perfect meal plan, along with timing. Although not conventional, I had her test her blood glucose to see if that played a role. Like with all my clients, we were looking for feedback.

Sara came back a week later. "I love this food, and I feel great!" she said. "The glucose monitoring kit is saying I have insulin spikes after grain and wine, though. What does that mean?"

Due to the response her body had, we focused on cutting out grains, limiting her wine, and not skipping meals. During our work together, she gained a few pounds and learned more about how her body processes food. This was important for her to be successful, and it's why it's key to not stick to one-size-fits-all plans when it comes to health.

As you apply the concepts in this book, keep in mind that we're figuring out your plan. Somethings may not happen the way you wished they would, but we have to let that go and give our body what it needs.

I know you can do this. You can figure out what you need, and how your body processes food or self-care or exercise or all the ways your body serves you every day. We'll get you to a better place together. I'm here for you.

Before we start creating the nourishing habits that work for you, I want you to understand *why* these habits actually serve you. All habits are multifaceted. In order to explain one habit, I may need to bring several scientific aspects into the discussion. I also want you to see that these habits are backed by science. As it turns out, nourishing our bodies is actually quite simple.

In the next part, we're going to review the science and stories I've gathered through the years to form these nourishing habits. Part Two is all about nourishing your body. Part Three goes into nourishing your soul.

You'll find each of the fourteen habits represented in the following chapters, with science-backed research that helps explain each one. I also use client stories to show you how these nourishing habits have changed lives and can change yours, too. Deeper explanations will help you understand the importance of these habits.

My hope is that the science and facts can provide an overview and motivation for you to make the necessary changes to your routine.

Let's start at the beginning, with how to nourish your body.

PART TWO

Nourishing YOUR BODY

CHAPTER THREE

NOURISHING HABIT #1: PROTECT YOUR SLEEP

We tend to sabotage our sleep with phones, TV, computers, and not going to bed early enough. Even foods like wine or chocolate have a big effect on how deeply and restoratively we sleep at night. Women that I work with tend to crave wine and chocolate most in the evening as a way to wind down, but these can actually key our body back up and throw off our sleep rhythms. Instead of helping us relax, they can prevent deep sleep, which only makes the cycle worse later!

Sleep plays a vital role in good health and well-being throughout your life. Getting enough quality sleep at the right times can help protect your mental health, physical health, and quality of life.[1]

Sleep also helps your brain work properly. While you're sleeping, your brain is preparing for the next day. It's forming new pathways to help you learn and remember information. Sleep is involved in healing and repairing your heart and blood vessels. Ongoing sleep deficiency is linked to an increased risk of heart disease,[2] kidney disease, high blood pressure, diabetes, and stroke. Sleep deficiency also increases the risk of obesity![3] You can be sabotaging your weight loss efforts simply by not letting yourself sleep.

Restorative sleep reduces stress, improves your memory, helps weight loss, and may help prevent cancer.

Insulin While You Sleep

Sleep also affects how your body reacts to insulin, the hormone that controls your blood glucose (sugar) levels. Without enough sleep, our blood sugar is higher than normal, which may increase the risk of diabetes.[4]

When your insulin is functioning well (partially thanks to getting enough sleep), fat cells remove fatty acids and lipids from your bloodstream. This is what we want because then the fat isn't stored. This impacts our weight, overall health, and cardiovascular health as well.

When you become more insulin resistant, fats or lipids circulate in your blood. This, in turn, pumps out more insulin, causing fat to be stored in all the wrong places, such as tissues like your liver. Although it may not seem fair, the more fat cells you have, the more likely you are to gain weight.

This is exactly how you end up suffering from diseases like diabetes.

Sleep and Weight Loss

Many people believe that hunger is related to willpower and learning to control the call of your stomach, but that's incorrect.

Hunger is controlled by two hormones: leptin and ghrelin.

Leptin is produced in your fat cells. The less leptin you produce, the more hunger you feel. But there's another hormone at play called *ghrelin.* The more ghrelin you produce, the hungrier you feel. Ghrelin also reduces the number of calories you burn (your metabolism) and increases the amount of fat you store. The more fat cells you have on your body, the more ghrelin you release.

Sleeping less than six hours a night triggers the area of your brain that increases your need for food, while also depressing leptin[5] and stimulating ghrelin.[6] In other words, you need to control leptin and ghrelin to successfully lose weight, but sleep deprivation makes that nearly impossible. This gets complicated because too little leptin makes you hungry, and too much ghrelin *also* makes you hungry.

When you're sleep-deprived, ghrelin and leptin are both affected, making it almost impossible to manage your appetite cues. If you stay up late and get up early, have young kids, or work night shifts, chances are good that you have a ghrelin-leptin issue thanks to lack of sleep.

You want to lose weight? Get more sleep.

Boosts Your Immune System

Your immune system relies on sleep to stay healthy because that's when it can best defend your body against foreign or harmful substances.

Ongoing sleep deficiency can change the way your immune system responds to common colds or bacteria. Sleep helps fight common infections[7] and is involved in healing and repairing the heart and blood vessels. When we get enough sleep, it reduces inflammation[8] and can slow aging. Our body uses sleep to rest and repair our tissues, which means we are better prepared to fight off illness and feel our best.

The Effect of Caffeine on Sleep

Four months before I met my client Marie, she had lost her husband to an incurable disease. In her grief, she had been turning to coffee, wine, and food to numb her daily pain. Because of all these sleep disruptors, her quality of sleep dropped, as well as the number of hours she slept. Gradually, instead of getting the eight or nine hours she needed, Marie's staggered sleep was broken up by frequent night wakings and a narrowing window of overall sleep time.

When we started working together, I made a few simple suggestions that would help her improve her sleep. "Stop eating earlier," I said, "and cut the coffee. Let's start there." Although my suggestions didn't seem to have anything to do with her sleep, she trusted me and went into action that week.

Once she stopped numbing her pain with food and cut out the coffee, her sleep began to change. It deepened, lengthened, and her health started to restore. Not only is she sleeping better now, but she's motivated to take overall better care of herself too.

Caffeine should be limited (all the time, but particularly toward the afternoon and evening) because it's a stimulant. Eventually, all stimulants become depressants because they deplete serotonin. Not to mention their profound effect on our sleep.

The only time I caution against limiting caffeine is if your adrenal glands are burned out. Try green or black tea so your sleep (which will ultimately help heal you from adrenal burnout) isn't so drastically affected. Work with your naturopathic doctor to determine if you have adrenal gland burnout.

Getting Better Sleep

Being a protective warrior for your sleep starts in the daytime hours before you lay down. Make sure you don't have too much caffeine, lower your lights, stay off social media, and let yourself wind down after dinner.

Melatonin is a hormone that helps us fall asleep at night. It's known as the "hormone of darkness"[9] because it's released due to a dark environment. When you create a dimmer environment at the end of the day, and you sleep in a dark room at night, melatonin is released to help you fall asleep. There is even early evidence that melatonin restrains cancer growth.[10]

If you need more help falling asleep, consider taking some supplements. Magnesium and potassium tend to help people sleep better. I started adding magnesium to my nightly routine, and it's worked for me. If you do nothing else to improve your sleep, try taking magnesium or eating more veggies with magnesium, like spinach, avocados, and nuts. Sleep masks can help shield light from your eyes when you're winding down, especially if you wake up in the middle of the night. You don't have to wear them all night.

Glycine is a lab you can have drawn through your naturopathic doctor that will tell you more about your sleep. For clients of mine that struggle with sleep, I recommend getting this feedback so they know if this is a problem for them. Glycine is an amino acid that can mess with sleep when glycine levels are low, and people with chronic sleep issues tend to have low glycine.[11]

L-theanine is an amino acid that helps with anxiety and better sleep. It's my personal favorite to help me sleep at night, and it can help anxiety during the day. You can also try 5-HTP, which stands for 5-Hydroxytryptophan. This amino acid is naturally produced by your body and helps you slide into a deeper sleep by increasing your production of melatonin[12] (amongst other benefits). It's also used as an appetite suppressant during the day.

There's also an herbal supplement called cortisol manager that has helped my clients with adrenal issues. Cortisol manager helps you get into a deeper sleep if you wake up in the middle of the night, thereby helping resolve the adrenal issues through rest.

CHAPTER FOUR

NOURISHING HABIT #2: DRINK WARM WATER WITH LEMON

The Detoxing Effect of Lemon

When I start working with a client, one of the first changes I have them make is to start drinking warm water with lemon every morning. It's a simple, quick habit to fall into that doesn't take a lot of forethought or preparation.

Water is amazing for you first thing in the morning because it keeps you hydrated, improves your skin, keeps your urinary tract healthy, reduces feelings of hunger, boosts energy, protects your vital organs, and can help prevent kidney stones.

Lemon can also help slow down our food absorption by aiding digestion. It also contains vitamin C, which is good for our immune system. Not only that, but the high amount of citrate in lemons can help protect against kidney stone development.[13] Studies have also found that lemon intake, combined with daily walking, can aid blood pressure management.[14]

Another great reason to have lemon in your water is that it gives your water a little zing. For some of my clients, it's helpful to have more taste in their water to keep them motivated to drink it.

A lot of the beneficial nutrients are found in the lemon rind, leading some people to zest the rind into their water as well. Try all these different methods, and find which you prefer. It may be a combination of them, which can help keep things interesting!

CHAPTER FIVE

NOURISHING HABIT #3: DRINK 8-10 GLASSES OF WATER PER DAY

Water is key to success with health, which is why two of the first three habits I want you to start creating revolve around water!

In general, we aren't getting enough water in our diets. The average person needs eight to ten glasses per day, but most of us are only drinking three to four glasses per day.[15] (If you're an athlete or really active or live in a hot climate, you may need even more.) Even if we hit our intake for the day, only about 30% of our water intake is actually water—the rest comes through soda, juice, and other less-healthy drinks. Unfortunately, when we are dehydrated, our body craves food first, not water. Your body *will* seek out food when it's thirsty, typically leading you to overeat in order to get more liquids from your foods.

If you're feeling thirsty, that means you're already dehydrated. A lot of our cravings and snacking issues can be solved by just grabbing a bottle of water and having a drink before we start to snack.

Drinking water can help flush metabolic waste products and

environmental toxins out of your body, promote feeling full, relieve back and joint pain, improve digestion, and help control your body weight.

Drink Quality Water

Water is a critical nutrient and essential for life, so we want to make sure we're drinking the *best* water. All kinds of contaminants can leak into our water systems, including nitrates from nitrogen-based[16] pesticides and pathogens like arsenic or illnesses.[17]

The EPA & EWG report[18] contaminants in water like nitrogen, bleach, salts, pesticides, metal toxins produced by bacteria, and human or animal drugs. There are biological contaminants as well, such as bacteria, viruses, parasites, and others.

When you drink water, make sure you know where it's coming from, that the quality is high, or invest in a good filter. If you aren't sure what's in your water supply and want a water filter, I highly recommend the Berkey system. They're reasonably priced and can last from anywhere between 3,000-6,000 gallons.

I also tell all my clients to avoid plastic bottles. Contaminants like BPA (Bisphenol A), microplastics, and others can leak into our water through the bottles. Research has linked BPA exposure to fertility problems, male impotence, and heart disease.[19]

Detoxifying

One of my clients brought her daughter, Paige, to see me because she had been gaining weight for the past few years. "Can you encourage Paige to eat healthy food?" she asked me. "We need some help there."

As we were talking, I noticed that Paige had acne and seemed to have very low energy. After I spent a while getting to know her habits, Paige said, "I don't drink much water, but I do exercise regularly. I also have terrible migraine headaches, and I'm constantly constipated."

These things had been going on for *years*. She didn't even know how to have a normal bowel pattern because it had been so long.

"Let's start by giving up caffeine," I told her, "and really focus on drinking more water. I'd like to see you have 8-10 glasses of water a day."

A week later, her mom called me. Paige had come downstairs screaming with excitement that morning.

"Her acne is going away," her mom said. "I can't believe it! She's having regular bowel movements. In fact, she's sometimes having bowel movements a few times a day! I can tell that she has more energy, and she's lost six pounds. Her migraines are almost gone!"

This success was a combination of her body ridding itself of toxins that had been sitting around for too long, causing her headaches and slowing her bowels. Increasing her water helped flush out those toxins, clear up her skin, and alleviate her migraines. Not to mention helping her bowels move more regularly again.

Sometimes, nourishing ourselves is as simple as grabbing a glass of water.

Diet Drinks

When my client, Sarah, came in to see me, she said, "I really only drink diet soda."

"Do you ever have water?" I asked.

"Not really."

Her goal was to get healthier and lose weight. She didn't really cook much and ate a lot of convenient, fast foods.

"Diet drinks are toxic," I said. "When we drink all the chemicals in them, those toxins are stored in our fat cells. Sometimes, our body may add fat cells to protect our organs from these toxic substances as they build up. Let's start you on the path to greater health by adding some water."

Thankfully, Sarah was willing to try. Within a week, Sarah was carrying around a new, twenty-ounce water bottle and never went back to diet sodas again. She lost thirty pounds and started a daily walking regime.

Sarah knew that diet drinks were bad for her when we started working together, but when she heard the powerful science behind why they were bad for her body, she had the power to give it up completely. That's what I want for you.

Make Water Easy

There are so many ways to be successful when it comes to drinking more water. (Like starting your day with warm water and lemon!)

- Consider buying a refillable mug that you can carry around.
- Avoid drinking from a plastic cup.
- Carry a water bottle wherever you go.
- Order water or hot tea without sugar when eating out.
- Try a soda water with lemon or lime when out with friends.
- Drink 1/2 cup to one cup each hour during the day to

space it out; then it's not so overwhelming. You can drink a cup on the hour, or have a chart on your fridge that you can mark off.

- Put a written reminder on your fridge or mirror.
- Tack a sign on your fridge that asks, in bright letters, *Am I hungry, or am I thirsty?*
- Keep a cup by your fridge or sink as a visual reminder.
- Make it a challenge with other members of your family! Recruit them to also drink enough water, then see at the end of the day who did it.
- If you get bored, add a wedge of lemon, try water with ice, or drink tea. Stay away from soda and artificial sweeteners.
- Create a daily checklist with drinking 8-10 glasses of water as one goal.
- Track your water consumption on an app. Some may even serve you occasional reminders to drink if you haven't in a while.

CHAPTER SIX

NOURISHING HABIT #4: FAST TWELVE HOURS AT NIGHT

Fasting has recently gained a lot more attention in the media because advocates for intermittent fasting as a weight-loss strategy have cropped up everywhere. With good reason: there's definitely science and proof behind intermittent fasting. I also advocate for fasting, but not in the way everyone else is talking about.

Historically, fasting is nothing new. References to fasting date as far back as biblical times, and current religious and cultures still practice it today. The recent push in studies that have confirmed the benefits, however, *is* new.

The word *fasting* sometimes triggers fear in my clients. The thought of going without food can be scary and anxiety-inducing. I understand. But with education and easing into it, this is a powerful strategy that can change your life.

What is Intermittent Fasting?

Intermittent fasting is a way to establish better boundaries for *when* you eat food, not how much of it you eat. When you fast, you try to put your body into digestive rest by not eating food or drinks that would trigger the digestive process for a set number of hours. There are no "rules" in terms of how you do it. The only rule I have is that you listen to what your body needs, and act on that.

There are at least fifty combinations of fasting, but the most basic breakdowns that you may find often look like this:

1. 12 hours fasting / 12 hours eating (12/12)
2. 14 hours fasting / 10 hours eating (14/10)
3. 16 hours fasting / 8 hours eating (16/8)

When you intermittent fast, you leave an *eating window* open, which is when you consume all your food. For my clients, I suggest they start with the 12/12 protocol. That means you stop eating when you finish dinner, and you have breakfast no sooner than twelve hours later.

Here's an example:

7:30 p.m.: You stop eating dinner
9:30 p.m.: You go to bed
6:00 a.m.: You wake up and get ready for the day.
7:30 a.m.: You "break your fast" with a healthy, balanced meal.

When you look at the breakdown, you can see that it's probably not *that* far from what you already do because so much of the fast happens while sleeping. This cuts out late-night snacking and has some of my clients go a little bit longer in the morning than they did before eating breakfast.

Fasting as a nourishing habit is still effective even if the focus is tailored around 12-16 consecutive hours of not eating. Some of my clients structure their schedule so they only eat about eight hours a day. That's fine if it works for your body, which is something you'll want to test.

If your body is healed and not in an inflamed state (which you might see with adrenal fatigue or thyroid issues), an occasional 24-hour fast is fine. You may even notice extra weight release when you do it. But if you attempt it in times of high stress, or your body is struggling, it will have the opposite effect. Women should only do extended fasts no more than two to three times per week, but I would advocate for even less.

One day, while visiting my client (who lives across the street) she mentioned she was doing a sixteen-hour fast. While talking in her kitchen, she reached into the fridge, pulled out some creamer, and poured it into her coffee—unbeknownst to her, creamer *will* break your fast!

She admitted that her body was not handling sixteen hours of fasting all that well. That time of year was particularly busy for her, and outside stressors made fasting more difficult. We moved her back down to fourteen hours, and then she tested how it felt for her. Based on her experiment, we realized that the additional two hours were stressing her body out. Once she went back to fourteen, her body was able to release some weight.

Weight Loss with Intermittent Fasting

Closing your eating window, and preventing blood sugar spikes late at night that interfere with sleep patterns, is an obvious way to help aid weight loss efforts. In fact, a study of 448 people who routinely fasted exhibited lower weight, lower fasting blood glucose levels, and fewer incidences of diabetes.[20]

Of course, correctly using intermittent fasting as a tool is the key. Although studies[21] have shown that women have a greater likelihood of losing fat and weight when using intermittent fasting as a nourishing habit, there is a way to take it too far.

In the intermittent fasting world, many people are doing extended fasts, sometimes for as many as twenty days. During that time frame, they only consume things that won't trigger digestion, like clear liquids and water. That is way too long! Going even twenty-four, thirty-six, seventy-two, or more hours without food can damage our bodies, especially for women. Extended fasting can change our hormones (particularly cortisol, the stress hormone, and adrenaline) and put us out-of-whack.[22]

If we're fasting for at least twelve hours[23] at night (aside from water), then our body has a chance to burn stored fat for fuel. When you venture over 12-16 hours, the benefits get a bit murky, especially for people with thyroid or blood sugar issues, hypoglycemia in particular.

For some people, an occasional 24-hour fast can be beneficial, but I only recommend this strategy for those who aren't in an inflamed state, feel motivated to do so, and ease into it slowly instead of all at once. If you fast too long and trigger a stress response, you'll bring your health backward a step.

Other Benefits from Intermittent Fasting

Intermittent fasting can improve more than just our blood sugar and weight loss efforts. Early studies in mice are showing massive effects on the brain from intermittent fasting, including possibly helping reduce the chance of diseases like Alzheimer's.

Here are some additional, research-backed benefits you can expect for your brain health from intermittent fasting:[24]

1. Intermittent fasting is proven to prolong the health span of the nervous system and may protect our neurons against genetic and environmental factors.
2. It increases cellular stress resistance, as well as reduces oxidative damage.[25]
3. Improves brain function.[26]
4. Possibly slows cognitive decline.[27]

Additionally, intermittent fasting affects our body right down to the cellular level. In our cells, the mitochondria are the powerhouse. We derive our energy because of our mitochondria. When we intermittent fast, particularly for fourteen to sixteen hours, it helps build up our mitochondria.[28]

It's also going to make you younger. The anti-aging effects of intermittent fasting come about because our body isn't working to digest all the time. It gives us the opportunity to repair and heal, which is where our inner maintenance man comes into play.

The Maintenance Man Visual

To help illustrate the benefits of intermittent fasting, I like to give my clients what I call *the maintenance man visual*.

Imagine a little maintenance man in your body repairing your cells, cleaning your arteries, and getting rid of toxins. He only works when we're sleeping, and he can only use stored fat as fuel. If we feed ourselves late night alcohol, food, dessert, or meals right before we go to bed, our maintenance man stops repairing and cleaning in order to process the food. Our body loves digestive downtime!

Think of it this way—you're either building your body up or tearing it down. And we know that our body always wants homeostasis. If we're tearing the body down, we need to build it back up. For women in menopause, your body is only in tear-down mode. (I swear, at fifty, it often feels like the Universe is trying to kill you off!) It's just one more reason that nourishing habits are so important.

A Few Considerations:

1. When fasting, tighten your eating window to eight or ten hours. You aren't restricting time *and* calories.
2. Don't rely on just black coffee to get you through. It expands in your gut and makes you think you're full when you really aren't, which can create problems later in the day.
3. If you're considering a 24-hour fast, think of the state of your body right now. Are you healed and healthy? Do you struggle with blood sugar, food cravings, or fatigue? If so, start slow, with fewer hours.
4. A 12- to 14-hour fast is ideal. Don't feel pressured to do more, but if you're feeling good and healthy and not stressed, you can try an occasional 16-hour fast.

CHAPTER SEVEN

NOURISHING HABIT #5: EAT THREE MACRO-BALANCED MEALS A DAY

When Cassandra and I met, she didn't really eat. At least, not in an organized manner. At sixty-five, Cassandra had a full and busy life, but she rarely made time to eat a healthy meal. "At thirty years old," she told me, "this was much easier! But my body doesn't seem to handle the day as well anymore."

Thanks to being an only child with a single mother, her habits had her reaching for fast food instead of fixing meals. A quick breakfast of coffee and pastries or whatever she could grab would lead into her busy day. By the time the afternoon rolled around, it had been six or seven hours since her last meal. At that point, she'd feel ravenous.

My first work with Cassandra included a discussion about the hormones of eating and how they can impact our day, our evening, and our weight. The education on ghrelin and leptin helped her understand what was happening. Once she knew that not eating three meals could cause hormone issues, she decided to make her first nourishing habit revolve around eating three meals a day.

Instilling the nourishing habit did not come easy at first. Cassandra and I worked through other habits to support eating three meals a day, such as planning and meal prepping. (She plans her day, including her meals, and takes food with her to eat now instead of relying on fast food.) In the end, however, the habits stuck.

She continues to enjoy better energy and better health, thanks to giving her body what it needs, when it needs it.

Eating three meals a day certainly helped Cassandra, but the greatest power truly came from the balance of fat, fiber, and protein she achieved as well. The importance of eating whole, fresh, organic, unprocessed foods that include a variety of fruits and vegetables cannot be overstated. That's why I encourage eating three macro-balanced meals a day as a habit you constantly repeat.

Fruits and veggies provide antioxidants, which fuel our immune system and keep us healthy. Protein helps us build muscles and stay fuller longer. Women also need to consume at least twenty-five grams of fiber a day—which isn't as easy as it sounds! One way you can hit that goal is through paying careful attention to your macronutrients.

Balancing your macros doesn't mean you have to count calories; it's simply a way to strive for getting all the right pieces in. Each of your meals should include a protein source, a fat source, and a low-carb, fibrous vegetable. For example, don't load up on one food group or a big plate of chicken or ribs. Balance that out with some salad and olive oil. Instead of eating just fruit, make sure you have protein and good fats. Have a little bit of everything on your plate. As a general rule, I encourage all my clients to focus on a green veggie, some protein, and a healthy fat.

The *macro* (meaning large) nutrients are fats, carbohydrates, and proteins. Here is a breakdown of what the macronutrients are, and why they get their own nourishing habit.

The Macronutrients
Fat

In 1976, Senator George McGovern from South Dakota raised a warning flag about the link between heart disease and high-fat diets during a senate hearing. In that decade, eight senators had died of heart disease, and people wanted answers. It felt like they were *dropping like flies,* and the American diet was suspect.[29]

From that hearing, the original American dietary guidelines were formed: we were told to eat less fat and more carbohydrates. Unfortunately, they didn't really have all the data. The science supporting it wasn't strong. In the end, this sparked a dieting craze that would eventually make American's fatter, incite fear of dietary fat, and change the landscape for heart health entirely.

Through bad research, fat was villainized as *the problem* with obesity, which meant that grocery aisles proliferated with fat-free options. Fat all but disappeared from grocery stores. Even the government supported further campaigns against it. I remember eating low-fat Snackwell cookies with my girlfriends and saying, "I'm so excited these are so good for us!" Unfortunately, that wasn't right!

Once we were told to fear fats (saturated fats in particular), we can look back and see a shift in the food industry. Serving sizes became huge. The fat-free craze led to a spike in the amount of sugar in all foods. Without any fat, nothing tastes good, so sugar came in as a quick replacement. Food companies even put additives in fat-free products to get you to eat more.

Look at society now—what happened?

American's became more obese than ever. Heart disease, diabetes, and extreme obesity proliferate. If you look back into the fifties, even in the movies, you don't see the rampant obesity that we have today. The fat phobia that arose after the fifties certainly hasn't made us healthier.

Our brains also need fat just to function,[30] not to mention that consuming healthier fats is a gateway to weight loss. Let's go into the protective effects of healthy dietary fat.

Fat Protects Us

Healthy fats are really good for our body. In fact, fat protects us. Sixty percent of our brain is fat,[31] and studies have shown that healthy fats can help prevent diseases like Alzheimer's.[32]

Fat is basically like a sponge that holds on to toxins, hormones, and vitamins[33] to use later when the body runs low or needs energy. In fact, the body stores all kinds of chemicals and pollutants in our fat cells, which can help protect our organs too. Every time you release unwanted fat cells, you are literally detoxing at the same time.

The more fat cells we have, the more estrogen is stored as well. A higher lifetime exposure to estrogen may increase our breast cancer risk.[34]

The Types of Fat

There are many types of dietary fat, and information can become confusing. Here are a few definitions:

Triglycerides: This is the main term for fat and fatty acids in our body, which breaks into two categories: *saturated* fat and *unsaturated* fat.

1. **Saturated fat:** When it comes to fats, you'll often hear them referred to as *saturated* or *unsaturated*. That terminology goes back to chemical and molecular structure. Simply put, a saturated fat is a type of fat that is typically still solid at room temperature. A few examples are butter, cheese, coconut oil, and red meat. These are typically more animal-based products.
2. **Unsaturated fat:** These fats are more likely to be a liquid at room temperature (like olive or avocado oil) and have heart-protective properties. These tend to come from more plant-based products. Unsaturated fats break down into two types: *monounsaturated* and *polyunsaturated*.
   a. **Monounsaturated:** The name derives from its chemical structure, but in general, monounsaturated are the healthy fats, such as olive oil, avocado, almonds, etc.
   b. **Polyunsaturated:** These fats can reduce cholesterol and lower your risk of heart disease or stroke.[35] Walnuts, flaxseed, and salmon are high in polyunsaturated fats.

Of course, this information can be overwhelming when we focus too hard on every detail, which is why I tell my clients to include the *healing* or *nourishing* fats on their macro-balanced plates. Healing fats include whole eggs, avocado, nuts, wild salmon, chia seeds, extra virgin olive oil, and dark chocolate.

One of the cooking fats I recommend is coconut oil. It is rich in fats called medium-chain triglycerides (MCTs), which are more fulfilling than others and can boost metabolism slightly. Coconut oil contains MCTs, which are easy to use and digest. Studies have also used oils containing MCT with Alzheimers or dementia patients and seen improvement. They can also help with weight loss.[36]

Of course, the brain needs fat, but we also need to have regulation. Too much saturated fat can cut off blood supply to the brain, which destroys neurons and also hardens arteries.

The Skinny on Fish Oil

When you take fish oil supplements (or you eat fish, walnuts, and ground flax seeds), you're supplementing your body with omega-3 fats. Omega-3's from marine-based fat sources (like fish) are fuel for our structural cells and brain cells.

Omega-3 breaks down into three different fatty acids:

1. DHA
2. ALA
3. EPA

DHA and EPA are mostly found through fish (you can consume ALA through plants and vegetables). DHA and EPA are important for your heart and linked to lower rates of heart disease. Eating fish rich in DHA has been shown to slow the progression of Alzheimer's disease.[37]

If you aren't already taking a medical-grade, high-quality fish oil, I encourage my clients to invest in their heart health with these easy-to-take supplements.

Carbohydrates

Years ago, while driving my daughter and her friend Sophie to a birthday party, Sophie said, "I don't eat carbs, to my daughter."

Startled, I looked at her in the rearview mirror. Surely, this was something she overhead from her mom. At a stoplight, I turned around in the seat and asked, "What do you mean?"

Sophie shrugged. "I don't know. I just don't eat them."

This random fact led to a conversation about carbohydrates. Despite her young age, this sentiment isn't unheard of. Lots of women rarely eat carbs. They're a hot topic right now thanks to the resurgence of low-carb diets like the ketogenic diet (consuming less than 20-25 grams of net carbs per day). The truth is that, like fats, not all carbs are created equal.

Carbohydrates are beneficial, just like fats. We shouldn't fear them or hate them either. Carbohydrates hold on to our electrolytes, making it easier to stay in homeostasis, and they give us fiber, nutrients, and vitamins. You also don't need grains to have carbs. Carbohydrates can come from vegetables and fruits. The vegetables and fruits that have carbohydrates also provide antioxidants that fuel our immune system to fight disease and keep us healthy.

When it comes to carbohydrates, I tell my clients to pay attention to what their blood glucose (or energy level) is doing and see how carbohydrates feel in their body. We don't want to over-consume carbohydrates, spike our blood sugar and insulin, and disrupt our energy levels. You'll know you're spiking your blood sugar if you feel energy for a while after eating, then crash and need a nap, more sugar, or caffeine to get through the day.

Not only does our body store excess glucose as fat, but too many carbohydrates raise our blood sugar and predispose us to diabetes.

Fiber is also an important aspect of the macronutrients we need (although some people don't count it as a macronutrient). Not only can it decrease our risk of colon cancer, but fiber (like in ground flaxseed and chia seeds) can absorb things like excess estrogen, bad cholesterol, and toxins. This helps to eliminate those things out of our body more easily.

Protein

With the current focus in nutrition revolving around various ratios of fat and carbohydrates, protein is sometimes overlooked. The importance of eating enough protein cannot be overstated. Protein has been shown to boost metabolism by burning eighty to one hundred calories more per day. It helps build our muscle and replenish our body after our workouts, which helps us maintain our muscle mass . . . and even increase it. Protein is essential for building our body back up.

My client, Amy, had been working out for years. She was thin, but not building muscle. "I want to make sure I'm healthy," she said at our first appointment. "Can you help me figure out how to be more defined and toned?"

After looking at her three-day food log, the problem became immediately apparent. She was not eating enough protein or calories. In fact, she wouldn't eat for hours after a workout.

"Let's add a protein smoothie after each workout after you do weights," I said.

Within a month, that toned look happened.

If we're not eating enough protein while working out, our body will take what it needs from our muscles. That isn't very productive! Excessive exercise without replenishing your body means your muscles will struggle to grow. If you're lifting weights, in particular, be sure to pay attention to your protein intake, and try to consume high-quality protein after a workout.

Try to find high-quality protein, preferably grass-fed, free-range meats like beef, poultry, and fish. Make sure they weren't fed corn or soy because that can dramatically affect the quality of meat. Of course, not everyone likes to eat meat. About 15% of my clients don't eat any meat. If that's you, turn to other sources of protein like beans, legumes, and nuts.

Soy as a Protein Source

Tofu (which is soy) is an option for protein as long as it's fermented, organic, and tempeh. Tamari is OK, as well as miso tempeh.

Be aware of soy lecithin, also. Soy lecithin is found in almost all chocolate (unless marked as soy-free) as a stabilizer. It's an oil extracted from soybeans by the chemical solvent Hexane, which isn't regulated. In general, soy is almost always genetically modified. It's hidden in a lot of things, too. Vegetable oil, for example, is really just soy.

Edamame is another form of soy that a lot of people turn to for protein. If you enjoy having edamame as an appetizer at a restaurant, for example, go for it! Just don't have it all the time, and understand that it's not the best form of protein for you. When possible, go for organic edamame.

Micronutrients

Nourishing yourself is all about feeding your body with nutrients, regardless of whether those are macronutrients or micronutrients. A lot of people think you just need to eat salad or lettuce, but that's not enough. When we eat crappy food or are struggling with cravings, we're usually starving for nutrients.

Micro (small) nutrients aren't needed in the same larger quantities as macronutrients, which we need in larger amounts. If we're focusing on the right macronutrients, micronutrients will follow. Examples of micronutrients include calcium, iodine, iron, potassium, magnesium, folate, zinc, and vitamins A, D, E, and K[38] (amongst all the others). We cannot produce our own micronutrients within our body, which means we need to consume them from high-quality food sources.

One way to ensure you absorb the micronutrients you need is by taking a probiotic. They help clean out the gut and also ensure that your body absorbs the nutrients, which helps you use the food you consume.

When you eat within the nourishing habits I've established and balance the macros on your plate, the micronutrients will show up.

Food Quality

Pay attention to the quality of the food you buy. Thanks to poor farming practices in our country, we often times have bad soil quality. That creates a problem with our food, which tends to be lower in nutrients. Supporting sustainable farming (which is soil that is still intact or rich with nutrients, so the soil is not depleted of minerals), can help us turn these practice around.

Trying to find food that is grown in nutrient-dense soil and is organic, synthetic, and pesticide-free can help maximize nutrient effects. Pesticides are chemicals that are sprayed on foods or put in the seed to ward off insects and bugs, but they can also affect our bodies. Some of my clients worry about the price of organic foods, which is usually a little higher. If you can afford it, do your body a favor and buy organic.

Think of organic, local, pesticide-free food as a type of health insurance! If you shop at a local farmers market and purchase what's in season at your grocery store, you'll find that the produce is much more affordable. It's often the same price as the non-organic produce.

When it comes to truly nourishing yourself, creating nourishing habits will help you get all your macronutrients, micronutrients, and create an environment where your body can optimally perform every day.

CHAPTER EIGHT

NOURISHING HABIT #6: KEEP YOUR INSULIN DOWN

When it comes to being our healthiest self, insulin is often an underestimated player in the game. Many of my clients come to me with an insulin issue, one that can't always be diagnosed through blood tests. When insulin levels go down, fat has an easier time getting out of the fat stores. That's when the body starts burning fat instead of carbohydrates.

Put simply, lowering your insulin puts fat loss on autopilot.[39] Your body becomes efficient at burning stored fat between meals and while you are sleeping. You will notice that you're not craving foods, especially carbohydrates.

Sugar

Sugar hides in everything.

This sneaky sweetener is in more than just candy. If you don't eat chocolate or sweets, that doesn't mean you don't take in a lot of added sugar. Sugar hides in bread, fruit, beans, yogurt, condiments, and more.

Not only is it snuck into almost everything, but manufacturers use different names for it, like brown sugar, corn sweetener, corn syrup, dextrose, fructose, glucose, high-fructose corn syrup, honey, lactose, malt syrup, maltose, maple syrup, molasses, raw sugar, and sucrose. Reading food labels—and knowing what they really mean—is key to success in identifying what is *really* in your food.

For example, let's say you're at the grocery store, walking around, and someone is sitting at a table. You get excited—a free sample! While they tout a laundry list of health benefits from their food, you munch into it. It's surprisingly delicious and sweeter than you thought. You get caught up in this hot new miracle product and buy some at the store, ready to tell everyone about it.

But then you get home, have some more, and look at the back. You can't find the ingredients list. The health information is buried. Weird. Then you finally find the fine print and see that is actually has a lot of sugar—the name for sugar is simply masked by something else.

When it comes to foods, particularly anything packaged, I always say, *read the label*. Although touted as healthy, the manufacturer may put extra sugar in something to make it taste good.

Along the same vein, some companies turn to sugar substitutions to replace our usual table sugar, but even they can cause carbohydrate cravings. Most of them are toxic chemicals and aren't good for our bodies. In fact, some sugar replacements are known to cause cravings.[40] The only exceptions I recommend are honey, stevia leaf, and maple syrup in moderation.

In fact, a study out of the University of Texas is showing interesting new connections between sugar and certain types of cancer, which seem to need sugar as fuel to grow.[41] There's mounting research evidence of a strong link between added sugar intake and some cancers, not to mention many chronic diseases

Sugar in the Body

Understanding the way our body uses sugar is pretty simple: the body is only going to burn one energy source at a time. It goes first to glucose. (Using protein can happen, but under different circumstances), then fat. If you're feeding the body glucose, it will use up what it needs, then anything left over is sent to your muscles. If it's not used up there, the body will store it as fat for later.

If we're always consuming sugar, our body doesn't burn fat. Then, because we eat sugar in excess in most societies, it's forced to continue storing it. The current culture around food has been to eat every 2-3 hours. If you're ascribing to the low-fat, high-carb lifestyle that has been recommended for so long, that means you're taking in a steady flow of carbohydrates.

Now think of that advice in terms of insulin.

We eat breakfast, increase our insulin response (insulin is the fat-storage hormone, so when we release it, the body is ready to store fat), and just as it's starting to slow down, we have a snack. At the point when our body could have switched to using fat stores, we give it more sugar. We're pumping more glucose into our body when we don't need it. Our intestines don't have downtime, and we're not giving the body the opportunity to burn stored fat because we keep our insulin high.

Sugar also creates an insulin response, which goes like this:

1. You consume sugar.
2. It travels from your stomach and small intestine into your

bloodstream. You may notice more energy while insulin helps your body use it . . . but it doesn't last.

3. Eventually, your blood sugar declines.
4. You start to feel exhausted. Your energy flags. You can't stop yawning. (Sound familiar?)
5. Your body signals you to eat more sweets or fruit or bread (because they turn to sugar) in order to get your energy back up.
6. Repeat.

When this happens, you're not giving the body an opportunity to digest fat in between meals. The body is going to use sugar as fuel instead of fat, which means it's just going to send the excess sugar to the liver to be stored as fat. It's an endless roller coaster.

The recommendations for sugar used to be fifteen grams (or just under four teaspoons) per day. The average American eats twenty-two teaspoons of sugar per day, which is eighty-eight grams of sugar! Because sugar isn't required for health, they've stopped recommending any amount of sugar, and instead suggest that we cut back to avoid obesity.[42] Now there is only a recommended maximum amount: twelve teaspoons, which is still ten teaspoons under what the average American consumes.[43]

To give you some reference, the average candy bar has around thirty grams of sugar. Regular Greek yogurt has upwards of twenty-five grams of sugar. Even iced tea has up to thirty grams of sugar in twenty ounces. That's over the recommended amount per day, for one item—not to mention how much else you're eating in other sneaky foods like muffins, fruit juices, and more. Sugar is literally everywhere.

On an initial call with a new client, Michelle, I asked the question, "Do you consume any soda?"

"Yes," she said. "I drink a 44-oz regular soda in the morning on my way to work, another one in the afternoon, and then I'll have a 16-oz bottle before I go to bed at night."

Her average day led to a total of at least 100 ounces of soda, and it wasn't the diet kind. After getting off the call, I looked up her favorite soda and figured out the math. Since one teaspoon of sugar is four grams, and 100 ounces of her favorite soda was 324 grams, Michelle consumed eighty-one teaspoons of sugar per day. That's over one-and-a-half cups, and that didn't account for any sugar in her food.

On our next call, I mentioned this to Michelle. "Did you know that in 100 ounces of soda, you consume over one-and-a-half cups of sugar per day?"

Silence rang on the other end for a moment. "Really?" she finally asked, sounding stunned. "I had no idea!"

That very day she quit drinking soda, and nearly six months later, still hadn't had any.

Sugar in Wine

A larger number of my clients come to me as avid wine lovers.

"I just love to wind down at the end of the day with a glass of wine," many of them say. "It gives me something to look forward to and helps me settle in."

What many of those women don't know when we first talk is that sugar hides even in wine! Wine is rampant right now. It seems to be everywhere. When I get my nails or my hair done, I'm also offered a glass of wine!

There are many reasons to avoid wine (and we'll go into those later), and one of them is the amount of sugar that hides in that little glass. Not to mention that trying to lose weight while consuming alcohol is much more difficult. With all that sugar, also comes a lot of calories.

Candida

In diets that have sugar in abundance, I often see clients struggle with candida, which is a naturally occurring yeast found in our gut, skin, and mouth. With a healthy individual, there are only trace amounts of candida present. We always have it, but it's usually in balance with our other gut flora. High amounts of sugar, however, can cause the yeast to proliferate and cause other issues. You may have also heard of *thrush* (candida in the mouth) or a vaginal yeast infection (candida in the vaginal canal).

Unfortunately, candida thrives on sugar. If you eat a lot of sugar, or have recently been on antibiotics that wiped out your healthy gut flora, candida may have had the opportunity to grow out of control.

To make matters worse, candida makes you crave more sugary foods, because sugar fuels candida, and it wants more. It becomes a vicious cycle. Even if you don't hoard candy bars and soda, you can still have issues with candida in your gut.

Unfortunately, sugar shares many characteristics common in drug addiction.[44] People don't talk about food being an addiction, but it definitely can be! We use food for all kinds of things. To celebrate. To comfort. To keep us energized. To cope. Unfortunately, we have to consume food, or we'll die, which makes combating sugar tricky.

Signs of Candida

If you suspect you have a candida problem, here are a few things to watch for:

1. Cravings for yeast, breads, and sugar.
2. Constipation, nausea, vomiting, bloating, gas, diarrhea (it basically wreaks havoc on your gut).
3. You're tired often.
4. You have white discharge in your underwear (for women).
5. White coating on your tongue.
6. Belly fat.
7. Foggy brain.
8. Itchy anus.
9. Joint pain.
10. String-like stool.

If you suspect you may have a candida problem, start with a medical-grade, high-quality probiotic, and cut back on your sugar intake. It will be hard at first, but power through the first three to four days. Not only will this help restore your gut health, but also help keep your insulin levels down.

If you suspect you have candida and want to get rid of it, go off sugar completely, or cut back gradually. Give yourself at least 7-10 days without it, which will allow time for the candida to start dying off, although it could take up to six months to really be gone. It thrives on sugar, so we want to remove its food source.

It's hard to cut sugar cold turkey because of withdrawals. My recommendation is to gradually cut back over a week, then completely avoid sugar once you subdue those cravings. That will help you kill any candida and cut your cravings completely.

Insulin

As a general rule, we don't want our insulin levels to go too high or too low. It's important for our body that insulin remain level so we have consistent energy—and don't have to deal with sudden, ravenous cravings that make us want to eat everything.

A balanced diet with good macronutrients keeps our blood sugar stable so our insulin doesn't spike up and down. When your blood sugar crashes after insulin has taken away all the glucose into the cell to be used, you may find yourself reaching for food again to get more energy.

Yet another vicious cycle associated with sugar.

We can actually cause our body to become insulin resistant. This whole process starts in the cell. Because of bad lifestyle and diet choices, we cause damage within our cells. The damage, combined with high-stress living, adrenaline, and cortisol, can block the action of insulin, causing sensitivity and eventual resistance.

Issues like insulin resistance can pose a big problem to losing weight. I've worked with clients who are eating healthy and exercising but are so sensitive to carbohydrates that fruit alone is causing them to keep weight on.

Katelyn came to me as a mother of two young children. She had a toddler, a newborn, and an autoimmune disorder. She struggled with fatigue, postpartum depression, and mood swings. Despite a basically healthy, paleo-based diet where her main carbohydrate consumption came through fruit smoothies every morning and vegetables like butternut squash, her scale wouldn't budge.

"I think you have an insulin issue," I said to her. "Let's try cutting out the fruit, and see if we can get things moving."

Once she cut out fruit and focused on keeping her insulin down and controlling her blood sugar, the scale started to move. Her energy began to stabilize. This isn't uncommon for the women I work with. Why? Because some women are more sensitive to carbohydrates, and they need to test removing them for a while to see what happens.

Fruit is great! I'm not here to make it a bad guy. There are lots of micronutrients and fiber and good things in it. But if you have an issue with insulin, even fruit can be damaging. It can be worth removing it to test and see if it makes a difference in your day-to-day energy levels.

CHAPTER NINE

NOURISHING HABIT #7: WEIGHT LOSS

Most of my clients come to me wanting to lose weight. Maintaining families, friendships, or relationships, raising children, expanding our careers, all while trying to fit in all of our own desires and dreams, often leads my clients to gain weight while in the pursuit of their best life.

For people that have extra weight to lose, the benefits are undeniable. Sometimes just losing a few pounds can help us improve blood pressure, have better sleep, and improve heart health.

There are a few key concepts I review with anyone that I work with that help create the right expectations for their weight loss. We're going to review them in this chapter. If you stick with the nourishing habits in this book, you're probably already losing weight or vastly improving your chances of doing so.

Hunger Hormones

Part of losing weight is understanding the interplay of different hormones in your body. Knowing how your body works can help you set yourself up for greater success. Let's review the three main hormones that affect the way your body controls appetite, suppresses fat, and processes the food you eat.

1. **Insulin.** You already know about this chemical messenger from chapter 8, but let's do a quick recap here. Insulin plays many roles in our body, including interacting with the other hunger hormones. Insulin is our fat-storage hormone and pops up in response to increasing blood sugars. The more sugar you eat, the more insulin you use. This can lead to fat storage as well as energy crashes— neither of which help us lose weight.

2. **Ghrelin.** Ghrelin is the hormone that's released as a signal to tell our body we're starving. Think of ghrelin as the *on* switch. It helps regulate appetite and protect us if we've missed a meal. When ghrelin enters the situation, our appetite is something that we have a hard time controlling.

   For example, when your stomach is empty, it creates ghrelin as a signal for you to eat more food. Let's say it's time for lunch. You're getting hungry, but you feel pretty in control. You get busy and don't eat, so more ghrelin is produced. Pretty soon, your appetite gets out of control. Even when you have the best intentions, like eating at your favorite salad place, you may find yourself eating anything you can get your hands on.

3. **Leptin.** Leptin is a hormone that tells us we're satisfied, especially if we're eating fat. When we're eating foods full of fat, leptin shuts off our signal to eat more.

   Think of leptin as the *off* switch. Leptin turns off the urge to eat once you've eaten, especially when high-fiber, high-quality foods are consumed. You can have 1,000 calories of unhealthy food and still be hungry because it didn't contain good nutrients. With the right foods, you'll likely eat less, be more satisfied, and nourish your body better. One thing I want to emphasize here: appetite regulation is not a calorie thing! Our bodies want high-fiber foods, increased protein intake, and healthy fats.

Understanding what hormones are at play can help you navigate weight loss. By avoiding ghrelin (which comes from skipping meals, going too long without food, or ignoring hunger cues), we can be better receptive to our body and keep our hormones at normal levels.

The Ghrelin Monster

I normally always schedule time to eat lunch when I'm working at my office. I'll usually run home or bring something with me to work to eat. But on one particular day, I had booked clients back-to-back without a break, and there wasn't time for lunch, so I skipped it.

By the time I returned home for dinner, I was beyond hungry—right up to ravenous. The moment I arrived, I started food-seeking. At first, I had some almonds, then popped a few raspberries in my mouth with coconut cool whip. A spoonful of almond butter with chocolate chips came next, followed by a piece of turkey. By the time I was reaching for my next conquest, I stopped and said out loud, "What am I doing?"

Right there, in the middle of my kitchen, I wrote down everything I had eaten just to see what it added up to. Even though it wasn't bad food, it wasn't mindful at all, and I was curious what it would total. It equaled what I would have normally eaten for an entire dinner!

I knew exactly what had happened—my ghrelin hormone had taken over. Because I skipped lunch, ghrelin had been sending a signal to my brain that I was starving. At that point, it was pretty much game over.

(You can binge on healthy foods too, by the way. We can eat really healthy food, but just too much of it.)

Some studies suggest that we have some mental control over how ghrelin affects our appetite. There was a study done that I call the milkshake study.[45] The goal was to determine if we had any mental control over our ghrelin response. The study took male athletes and gave them all the same full-fat milkshakes. Half of them had a milkshake labeled *full fat* ice cream, and the other half had a milkshake that said *diet*. All the boys that drank the full fat milkshake were satisfied. The other group was still hungry afterward, which certainly suggests that we have some conscious control over ghrelin.

I like to have my clients talk to their ghrelin hormone, as crazy as it sounds. If you think you're deprived, you will be. Talk your way through that idea and into a calmer mental landscape. Sometimes, talking to your ghrelin can help!

For example, let's say a meeting went late, and it's 3:00 p.m. You're finally free, and you're *starving*. Instead of rampaging through a drive-through and eating the first thing you can, just stop. Talk yourself down a little bit.

Try something like this:

"I'm not starving. I'm just really hungry because I have too much ghrelin. My body is not starving. I am not in danger. Thank you, ghrelin, for protecting me, but everything is fine here."

You might be surprised what happens when you take a breath and allow yourself to be mindful. Plan your meals ahead of time to help prevent your inner ghrelin monster, and definitely, don't skip lunch. Then you have to fight the snacky, hangry ghrelin attitude at the end of the day.

A few important facts about ghrelin to keep in mind:

1. If you don't get enough sleep, you'll have more ghrelin.[46] This makes it harder to keep snacking and appetite under control.
2. Don't skip any meals! (Especially lunch.) When you skip meals, you produce more ghrelin, and it makes it harder to stay in control later.
3. The more fat you have on your body, the more ghrelin your body produces.
4. Responding to ghrelin creates an unfair, vicious cycle, because it often causes you to snack unconsciously, sneaking in food you didn't really need. Not only will that affect your health, but your other hunger hormones too. Snacking when you aren't hungry, or eating sugar to keep yourself awake, will cause an increase in insulin—and subsequent drop—which will only make you *more* tired later.
5. Keep twelve hours in between dinner and breakfast as a fast, but make sure you have a nutrient-dense breakfast. This helps keep the ghrelin monster under control during the day.

Dealing with Cravings

The bummer about cravings is that they exist, and they *definitely* affect our weight loss efforts.

Cravings can be like a tidal wave that crashes over us, especially because ghrelin comes into play. When we first start changing our habits and moving toward a nourishing lifestyle, we're typically much more careful about what we eat. That's because we're actually getting to know ourselves. We know that a brownie could trigger us and end in eating the whole pan. Or, one drink of wine, and suddenly the whole bottle is gone. However, the problem often arises with my clients when they've been consistent for a while in their new, nourishing habit.

Sometimes we just . . . get a little cocky; then we get sloppy. We think it's not a big deal (and it shouldn't be) if we veer away from our nourishing habits for a day or two. So we do.

We indulge for that weekend, that cheat meal, or that week of vacation. When we come back to reality, we're motivated to get back to our healthier plan again. Then the cravings hit, and we can't stop them. Our weekend off somehow becomes a week.

A month.

A year.

Suddenly we're back where we were before and more frustrated than ever.

There are many factors that affect our cravings, such as emotional attachments, stress, candida, and low serotonin levels. In fact, eating carbohydrate-rich foods cause an increase in serotonin, which has a mood-altering effect.[47] It makes us feel better. It's the same mechanism as nicotine. If our serotonin levels drop, our body will often trigger sugar cravings. Once that is consumed, serotonin levels increase again, making us feel "happier" for a brief time. Unfortunately, this also perpetuates and feeds an unhealthy cycle.

When we're in the midst of a craving, the strength of it can be shocking. *If I don't eat this,* we may think, *I'm going to die.*

You aren't going to die.

There's really only one way to stop your cravings: you just have to kill it. This is key. You cannot keep eating sugar and kill candida. Once you stop feeding it sugar, the body sends a distress/need signal (craving) that says you need sugar, *now!* Essentially, part of your body believes that last time sugar was taken in, it made everything better. (This is where those pesky serotonin levels come into play.) Don't feed it! That will only make candida and the cravings worse.

When cravings strike, I find that a pot of hot tea can be a lifesaver. My client, Katie, went through withdrawals when she stopped eating sugar for the first time. Once she decided to try it, she went cold turkey. Her body reacted with nausea and cold sweats before it transitioned out of the symptoms. In the end, she felt much better without it, but she had to work through the withdrawal first. This is normal for most women I work with.

You can cut back on your sugar gradually or all at once, whatever feels best to you. If you're cutting back gradually, just make sure that you eventually stop all sugar (or whatever you're craving) for at least seven to fourteen days. If you're used to eating a candy bar every day, let's instill a new habit.

You may feel some side effects from going off the sugar, such as:

- Fatigue
- Generally not feeling well

- Acne
- Moodiness
- Flu-like symptoms

These symptoms will pass. If you get rid of the craving entirely, then you have a chance to start something new and stay on that path. Otherwise, if you keep giving in to the craving, you end up white-knuckling through them all the time. That's a stressful place to be and certainly doesn't aid our overall health.

My client Monica traveled a lot for work as a sales manager. Her eating habits were pretty good . . . except for her love of treats. And Monica had a very real *thing* for sweets.

"I love eating treats, Julie," she said, her eyes shining. "They taste so good, give me something to be excited about, and make me happy when I'm indulging. I don't know if I can give that up."

"They do taste good," I said, "but let's work on balancing them out with some more nutrient-dense foods, and gradually cutting back. Give your body an opportunity to see what happens without them."

With some reluctance, she agreed. For the next week, we worked on balancing nutrient-dense foods and limiting her sugar. When she reported the next week, she said, "My body does feel different. I feel less inflamed, and my energy is better. I really can't believe it. Even though they taste good, this feeling is better. Sugar isn't good for me!"

After we celebrated her win, her voice sobered. "Here's the thing, though. I have a sales meeting coming up with my boss and the entire sales force. In the past, they've had an array of candy. It's their attempt to make things fun and get employees to participate. What do I do? I don't want to be rude, but I also don't want to go down that path again."

"You need a plan," I said. "We can do this, but if you plan for it, you'll be better prepared."

Together we came up with a plan. When Monica sat down, she'd move any visible candies to the side so she could get them out of her sight. If called upon, or asked whether she'd like one, she would say, "No, thanks!"

Monica called after the sales meeting. "Julie!" she sang, "It worked! I know it's because I went into it prepared with what I would do and say. I'm still off sugar and feeling better every day."

This brings us back to our nourishing habits. We put things into place to protect us so it's easier when we start to drift away or indulge in unhealthy cravings again. I don't mean to villainize certain foods—it's okay to treat yourself or not be 100%. We can't always live in a world of black and white. Having a plan and realistic expectation for after the treat will help you get back on track quicker.

Most of my successful clients are the ones who kill the craving and eventually stop having cravings at all—for wine, sugar, coffee, or anything else. Being in a place where you have no cravings is normal. Cravings are not normal. Get to that point so you can thrive on a balanced eating plan.

Comforting with Food

Sometimes we have to slowly wean ourselves off of the foods we have the hardest struggle with because we tend to use them as a sort of emotional crutch. When my clients are upset, or suddenly off track, or struggling to find motivation, I often ask, "What's eating you?" The responses are always revealing of deeper emotions or issues.

Food provides comfort, especially when we are tired, in pain, sad, or lonely. For most of my clients, it's easier to slowly limit these foods because the withdrawal is easier to deal with. Being aware that you're using food as a comfort is the first step. Then, you dive deeper the way I encouraged in the beginning and start asking *why?*

Why am I comforting with food?

Why am I feeling this way?

What has caused this?

Dive into the root of the problem instead of turning to that box of sugary donuts. You'll not only feel better because you ate nourishing food, but you'll work through the emotions that tend to eat *you*.

The Scale

When it comes to weight, the scale isn't always accurate.

So many things can mess with your daily weight, like water, bowel movements, extra sugar intake, and high sodium consumption the day before. Some women who come into my office notice inches are gone, but no weight has changed. Go by your inches and how your clothes feel, not by what the scale says. Weight loss is all mindset. If you don't have the proper mindset, it's not going to work.

Despite this, I sometimes encourage my clients to use the scale as a tool, just not the *only* tool. Inevitably, after my clients start building their nourishing habits, they gain great traction. Then something may happen. A family tragedy. A birthday party. A girls' night out where they drink more than they anticipated and then snack. During our conversations, my clients may often say, "I feel like I'm slipping off track," or "I'm losing momentum, help!"

This is when I advocate for the scale to come back as a means of tracking what's happening—but not as a source of shame. Watching what your weight is doing over several weeks can help you stay motivated, understand your body, or at least hold on to one habit when it feels like all others are slipping away.

Troubleshooting Weight Loss

Here are a few ways to troubleshoot if you're instilling all the nourishing habits we've spoken about, but still not losing weight.

1. Stop focusing on the scale alone. There is no failure on the scale, only feedback, so don't take one bad weigh-in as an indication of failure. That can drive us to emotionally eat, sabotaging our efforts.
2. If you've been tracking, look back over your log. What was different? What feedback can you find? Did you track honestly, or were you sneaking things in that you didn't record?
3. Celebrate victories away from the scale, like better fitting clothes, feeling more comfortable in your own body, sleeping more soundly, having clearer skin, or noticing an increase in your exercise stamina.
4. Measure yourself instead of using only the scale. Go for inches lost instead of pounds. I suggest that you measure hips, thighs, arms, and waist. Make sure you write down notes on where you first measured, so you go to the same

spot the next time. Do whatever schedule you like, but I suggest you measure every week. It can help you stay motivated and get a baseline.

5. If you have a bad weigh-in, always look back to the previous day. One little-known fact is that not drinking enough water the day before can affect your weight. Drink more to keep your body hydrated, which flushes sodium and toxins out.

6. Constipation can also affect weight. When did you last have a bowel movement?

7. Did you eat a salty meal the day before? Extra salt can cause you to retain water.

8. Give it time. If you've just made some lifestyle changes, it can take a while for that to work through your body. This is a good point to ask whether you should be stepping on the scale less. While I advocate for knowing your weight, I don't advocate for obsessing over it. Use the scale as an extra tool and don't be afraid of it.

9. I tell my clients that, "Your body wants to trust you." Sometimes the scale doesn't move because your body wants to trust you. Once it knows you're not doing something crazy, it tends to just release the weight. Remove the stress. Build your body instead of tearing it down, and give it time, but don't give up.

10. In the past, if you've eaten really low calorie to lose weight (less than 1200 calories per day) and are doing so now, make sure you bump those calories up. Reducing calories may not actually help long-term weight loss.[48] Increase

your calories, because it often helps the body release more weight. Once the body seems to be more secure, you're more likely to see change.

11. You don't have to work out a long time to lose weight! One study has shown that even eleven minutes of resistance training can accomplish a great deal of benefits toward your health and fitness.[49]

PART THREE

NOURISHING YOUR *Soul*

CHAPTER TEN

NOURISHING HABIT #8: GRATITUDE

The power of gratitude is undeniable.

Studies abound with references to the positive health benefits of gratitude. In fact, our ability to have gratitude in the moment may be central to our capacity to flourish.[50] Gratitude broadens our mind. It builds positive feelings of trust. It centers us in the moment and helps us be aware of what we have, which allows our body to release chemicals that have a positive effect on our body.

Gratitude is also a uniquely human trait—one we should take advantage of. We can appreciate what we have, even at a micro level, and create greater capacity for growth because of it.

Studies have also shown that daily gratitude lists help alleviate depression.[51] I know that if I'm feeling bummed, depressed, anxious, or not good about myself, I stop. Then I ask myself, "What do I have right now?" "What am I grateful for?"

My client Simone said, "I haven't lost weight as fast as I wanted. Everything seems to move more slowly than it used to before I had kids. Exercising isn't as easy, and I'm exhausted at the end of the day. I get really hard on myself and feel defeated, but I've also realized that I'm in better health than I used to be. I've made some progress. And then I realized I needed to be grateful for what I had, because not only am I moving in the right direction, but I have a beautiful family going there with me."

Having gratitude can help our outlook. Like anyone, there are times when I get scared, bummed, or start spinning around the *what-ifs* that may happen in the future. When I realize the *what-ifs* are causing me to spiral, I stop and say, "I'm not letting that fear rob me of today and all I have."

One way to look at it is this: a rip current versus the beach. When I'm in that bad place, I ask myself, "Do I want to overthink everything and 'swim in the rip current' or sit on the shore and let the thoughts come and go without investing my emotional energy into each one?" It's hard to live in the moment when you swim against the rip current.

At that moment, I'll open my phone, search for gratitude quotes online, go through each one, and keep reading until I feel better. It helps me come out of that funky place where we get so down on ourselves. It seems like one step into that funky place leads to a deeper one, and then suddenly we're eating ice cream out of the freezer.

Visualizing what you're grateful for, or what your ultimate goal is, can help you feel more gratitude as well. Visualizing your thoughts helps you paint a better mental picture, and breaks through your protective primal brain so you can actually achieve your goals or feel better about your current position. Taken in hand with gratitude, it's a powerful way to change.

My client, Amanda, called me one day, distraught. Through tears she said, "I don't believe I can do this, Julie. It's too hard."

"Amanda, you don't have to be perfect!" I cried. "Look how far you've come! Remember where you started. If you look back and have gratitude for what you've already done, it will help you focus on positivity."

Together, Amanda and I stepped back, reviewed where she started, and set her on a better path of gratitude.

Sometimes we focus on the things that we don't have, or we compare ourselves to the people we follow on social media (and think their picture-perfect world is real!). If we just stop and ask, "What do I have? What am I grateful for? My house. My car. My partner. My family." If we start with the basics, then the gratitude will calm that negative voice.

Plus, gratitude is so easy. We don't need anything to stop and be grateful. Even on our worst day, we can think of something to be grateful for. It's one of the best ways to truly nourish your soul.

Ways to Have More Gratitude

1. Look up inspirational quotes on gratitude or pictures with quotes on them.
2. Ask others what they are grateful for.
3. Help others in need. This is a firsthand way to see how truly lucky we are.
4. Make a list of everything you have.
5. Take an inventory of your life. Focus on the opposite of what you are complaining about.
6. Example—if you had to take a lower-paying job, say, "I'm so grateful that I have a steady flow of income and I have the skills to have gotten this job," instead of being angry. If you're stuck in a relationship, focus on what you get from the person not what you're *not* getting. Thank them for that thing.

CHAPTER ELEVEN

NOURISHING HABIT #9: SELF-CARE

Despite what most women tend to think, self-care is *not* selfish. In order to truly nourish your soul, you have to put yourself on top of your to-do list. This may be one of the most important nourishing habits you put into place, and also one of the hardest.

Being healthy is a lifestyle where you take care of yourself. That doesn't mean you have to do everything by yourself. Don't be the last person on your list. Some of my clients act more like a maid than a part of the family.

Shelly came into my office for one of our weekly check-ins with a vast list of things that she needed to do. "I just got off of work," she said, blowing in with a frazzled air. "I have to leave a few minutes early so I can drop my kids off, then I have to go to an event after I make dinner. I'll eat sometime after that because I have to run to the store."

Shelly gave her all to her work, church, after-hours meetings, events, and then to her family. In fact, she would often watch her family eat while she was doing something else, then eat by herself later that night. Of course, it's easy for us to stand back and see there are several problems with her habits, but when it's happening to us, it's so much harder to be self-aware. Shelly had no self-care or boundaries.

I want better for you. I don't want you to be frazzled or stressed or miss out on moments with your family. Don't live on the sideline. Go all-in.

Boundaries Are Self-Care

So much of nourishing ourselves revolves around setting firm boundaries, whether that means for work, relationships, or our own habits.

In my time working with Shelly, we did a lot of work around setting boundaries. "Do you want to be this busy?" I asked her. "Do you have to be this busy for financial reasons?"

Puzzled, she shook her head. "No."

"Which of these jobs feels fun to you? Do you feel rewarded by or energized from any of the things you do?"

"A company asked me to be on their board," she said, her expression dropping. "The long monthly meetings would totally drain me, but the president told me I was the only one for the job. They asked me, 'Don't you see this position is your calling?' My family and husband are already suffering from our busy schedule, not to mention my health. Taking this on would mean a lot more time away from my family and more stress."

"What do you think God is telling you?" I asked. "What is your gut telling you to do?"

After a little thought, she said, "I think God is calling me to be at home. This is my daughter's last year before college, and I don't want to miss that."

With gentle nudging, she politely declined the offer, freed up time so she could spend it with her family, and brought her stress level down. After setting that boundary, she felt great! She ate dinner with her family a little earlier, which helped her create a fasting deficit to help heal her body.

Another client, Tammy, has a hard time saying *no* when her daughter asks her to watch kids while she goes to the gym or out on dates. She feels bad because her daughter has been through a lot, and Tammy doesn't want to be selfish. Tammy remains at home, caring for all the children, but never takes time for herself. Over time, this has become a big stressor for her. We don't have to have that stress in our lives! We can say *no*, choose ourselves, and set boundaries with those we love while still keeping the relationship intact.

It's great to help our family or friends, but when they stop asking, and make the assumption that you'll say *yes*, you may feel your life slipping away. Stop for a moment, create some boundaries, and allow yourself to find balance.

When we set good boundaries, we take care of ourselves.

> "Take care of your body. It's the only place you have to live."
>
> –Jim Rohn

The Self-Care Tank

When I flew to France with my daughter, I had *big* plans to get work done. "I'll have hours to fill while on the plane," I told myself. "I know I can get a lot done."

After boarding, settling in, chatting with my daughter, and taking off, I pulled out my computer. Then the screen on the back of the seat in front of me caught my eye, so I started to flip through the movie options. Minutes later, I found myself settling into the first of three movies. All my plans for getting work done slid away as I relaxed, laughed with the movies, and sank into the experience with my daughter.

For me, that day, it was the ultimate self-care.

I tell my clients that we have three tanks that need to be filled: the love tank, the happy tank, and the self-care tank. If you go get your nails done, your hair trimmed, sit down with a new book, or simply do *nothing* during your downtime, it fills up your tank! Downtime fills up our happy tank *and* our self-care tank so we can deal with all the other stuff that comes our way. There's something about having a little *me* time that makes it so things don't seem so hard.

"I normally push through everything," my client, Andrea, said. "Workouts, dealing with my day, getting my house cleaned, and powering through my list. Finally, one day, I decided to sit down when my legs started to ache instead of doing the dishes. I just watched a TV show, gave my body a chance to wind down, and did the dishes later. Nothing fell apart. In fact, I felt better. What I used to think was a sign of aging is really just my body saying it needs a little break every now and then."

Self-care comes back down to science. When we take care of ourselves, we get a little shot of happy in the form of serotonin (a neurotransmitter that works in our brain). Every time we do something to take care of ourselves, we're rewiring our brain to do *more* of that thing. Self-care strategies that are known to boost serotonin include sunlight, being outdoors, massage, exercise, laughter, and happy memories.[52]

Self-care doesn't have to be difficult. For example, the other day,

I ran to my doctor's office and accidentally left my phone at home. Instead of scrolling Instagram, I picked up a magazine on the coffee table and flipped through it. "Oh my God!" I said, laughing, "This is so awesome. I haven't looked at a magazine in forever."

While nothing huge, it was fun and silly. Tangible. I held it, flipped through it, and enjoyed doing a fun, unexpected thing. It gave me that little shot of happy that helped add to my self-care tank.

The best kind of self-care is sometimes spontaneous and relies on us to do it. Taking care of ourselves nourishes not only us, but all those that rely on us through our families, businesses, and lives.

Pity Parties

Cindy came in for our appointment one week and told me, "I'm hungry all the time."

At this point, she'd been coming to me for over a year. When we started working together, she only drank diet soda and no water. She didn't exercise and mainly ate fast food. Her weight loss had slowed down recently and I wondered why. Up to that point, however, she'd been doing a fantastic job.

"You're hungry all the time?" I asked, startled. In all our time together, she'd never said this before.

"All the time."

Further exploration revealed what was going on—she was having a pity party. One of those moments where everything seems out of control, or bigger than it is, and we just feel sorry for ourselves. This isn't necessarily a bad place, but I don't want you to stay there. Sometimes, it takes a little self-care to get us out of that place, gain some perspective, and back on our consistent plan.

If a pity party pops up, go with it for a few minutes, just don't move there. It will feel like you're fighting your body if you keep throwing a pity party for yourself. Veer back to that consistent path, and you'll see results, even if it doesn't feel like it at the time.

CHAPTER TWELVE

NOURISHING HABIT #10: POSITIVE SELF-TALK

When I first married Jack, I bought a book titled, "How to Have Confidence." I remember feeling embarrassed when buying it, hiding it under my arm while walking to the front of the store, like I was buying the karma sutra or something! *I don't want anyone to know I don't have confidence,* I remember thinking.

Wouldn't it be great if there were a *confidence button* we could push and suddenly feel good about ourselves? Despite being tall, thin, and well-liked, I didn't *feel* it was true. At times, I felt confident, but the feelings started to disappear in the folds of uncertainty that comes with life.

Maybe you are searching for that special *confidence button* too. Something that will teach you the secret of how to do it all and be it all. The truth is that you already have it all inside of you.

I believe that we are born with confidence. The encroachment of negative things through the childhood years can change our perception of ourselves and our confidence levels. Through all the trials of life, we have to decide who we want to be and figure out a way to make that happen.

In other words—we don't have to take in negative comments. We don't have to repeat them and invest in them. We can use them for feedback to push us, but it's important to keep a balance of giving ourselves grace and doing self-care at our own pace.

This all comes back to the way we talk about ourselves.

Some women feel like they're never going to win. I want to shake them and say, "You are so wonderful! Stop listening to the negative voice that says you won't succeed. Stop!"

We all have a negative voice that speaks inside us. Talk back to it! "No," you can say. "I am going to succeed. I'm working on myself. Any good things I put into place are going to affect my health positively. If I fall off the plan, that's fine. I don't want to be perfect. I'm going to give myself grace, the way I would for a friend."

Despite my embarrassment, buying that book on confidence was the moment when I realized I needed to change my mindset and the way I spoke to myself. Taking care of ourselves—nourishing our soul—is often about what we say to ourselves, not just what food we take in.

You hold your own power. Most of that power lies in the words that you say to yourself, oftentimes without realizing what you're saying.

Thanks to the nature of my work, I hear the things women say to themselves about their bodies, careers, addictions, and more. That's why, with all my clients, I work with them every week to make sure their self-talk is positive and not negative.

Negative Voice

All of us have a negative voice inside us, saying that we're not good enough, or we'll never succeed, or we don't deserve to be happy. When we go into our day, we often wake up feeling pretty good. Our stomach is flatter, we've had some rest, and we're ready to conquer the world. It often takes just one or two things to throw us off and into a negative spin.

We have to learn how to cheer ourselves on when we hear the negative voice that says, *you will never lose weight,* or *you will never be thin,* or *you are not good enough.* Oh, but you are good enough! You are great! You just have to keep telling yourself you are until you finally believe it.

Whatever you say to yourself is going to happen. Like my client, Leslie. "I've done this multiple times," she told me. "Part of me thinks that this isn't going to work. I've tried to change so much."

"You have to stop that mindset," I said. "You won't succeed if you keep saying you're not going to succeed."

Listening to what you're telling yourself and changing that negative voice to positive is the first step. When you hear yourself say, "This isn't going to work. It never has in the past, and it won't now," then stop. Give yourself a moment of gratitude, then change to a more positive thought. Try on these:

1. I am going to succeed with this plan.
2. I know I can do this.
3. This is so easy for me.

Maybe it doesn't feel honest or natural at first, but you can change the way you think and perceive yourself by switching to positive thoughts. That's why it doesn't matter what I tell people to eat, because we end up having to work on positive mindset no matter what.

In fact, studies have confirmed that the way we speak to ourselves can actually increase our self-confidence and performance levels and reduce anxiety.[53]

What My Clients Say to Themselves

1. This is so hard.
2. I can't do this.
3. I can't eat that.
4. I can't stand my body.
5. I'm lazy.
6. I'm fat.
7. This is going too slow.
8. Maybe there's something wrong with my genes.
9. Maybe there's something wrong with my thyroid.
10. What makes me think I can lose weight?
11. I'm a failure; I might as well eat this.
12. Diets are dumb.
13. I give up.
14. I'm never going to lose weight.
15. I hate to cook.
16. I'll start my diet tomorrow.
17. I messed up. I ruined it.

The Comparison Game

So many women come into my office with the problem of comparing themselves to other women. Often, when we see other women and what they have, we tend to compare ourselves automatically. I'm always telling my clients, "Don't compare yourself to anybody else!" It can undermine all our hard work and effort.

It breaks my heart to see so many of us trying so hard, but never feeling better. Running a business, taking care of a family, tending to those that need us, and having a life, is hard enough. Add in the pressures of social media, and sometimes we can get sucked into the comparison game without even realizing it.

We scroll through Instagram or Facebook and silently think, *look at what all these people have going for them. What about me?* Or, *I could never do that,* or *my business is definitely not that put together.*

We've got to stop.

Not only is it a time-waster, but it doesn't promote greater nourishment or belief in ourselves. Find a tribe of people you like, and stick with them. If you follow someone on social media that triggers this response in you, let them go! Unfollow those that don't cultivate positive feelings, and stop comparing. There's so much behind the scenes of their perfect life that we don't see. Staying positive comes more naturally when we aren't constantly comparing ourselves against a standard that doesn't exist outside our heads.

ANTS Syndrome

I've struggled with anxiety since I was little. Even as a small girl, I could lay in bed for an hour overthinking things, with my brain looping endlessly. My divorce from Jack certainly didn't help, nor did taking a chance by opening my own business. Through time, counseling, learning, and reaching out, I've been able to train myself to back away from the temptation to spiral. A lot of small things add up to big differences in managing my anxiety.

For example (and some of these may sound familiar!):

1. Not comparing myself to other people.

2. Having a higher power to tap into, whatever that is for you.
3. Prayer/Meditation.
4. Journaling.
5. Saying the opposite of something negative.
6. Working with a counselor.

As women, we're often spinning through the *what-if* and the *worst-case scenario* games in our head. Instead of asking *what if this bad thing happens,* ask *what if I'm meant to be here* or *what if this amazing thing happens?* For whatever reason, there could be a silver lining that will come out of a bad event, one that you didn't anticipate. Sometimes things are happening for us, not to us.

No matter how you look at it, anxiety is tied to our mindset and the way we speak to ourselves. This can have a direct effect on our mental state. One quote that I love demonstrates this perfectly. It says, "Living in the past is depression; living in the future is anxiety." So live in the moment! And enjoy it!

In fact, Dr. Daniel Amen calls it the *ANT Syndrome* (or ANTS—Automatic Negative Thoughts Syndrome).[54]

Anxious thoughts start off small, then grow. Lots of them tend to clump together. Before you know it, there are so many you can't keep track. You're looping on problems again and again. When we don't know the solution, and we're afraid, we end up thinking about all the things that could go wrong—which further paralyzes us. We create problems that didn't exist. This is ANTS working against us.

Of course, anxiety isn't always just about our mind. There are other factors that can affect whether we struggle with anxiety. For example, the microbes in our GI tract have a marked influence on our emotional state. Pathogenic gut bacteria can create an issue with anxiety and depression.[55]

My client had high copper when we had her blood work drawn, which can often manifest as anxiety. Copper imbalances can sometimes come from birth control medication. It can wreak havoc on our system and our gut and cause an imbalance that manifests through things like anxiety.

There can be a lot of underlying issues happening that cause ANTS. Instead of assuming that there's something wrong, getting bloodwork may show if you're deficient. Supplement imbalances play a key role here, even if they don't treat the entire issue.

As a society, we're almost 80% deficient in magnesium, which can absolutely manifest as anxiety or overthinking. Taking a magnesium supplement creates a calm environment in our body. I recommend you take magnesium at night to help your muscles relax so you can get more sleep and decrease anxiety as well. Low B vitamins can also contribute to anxiety. If you don't process folic acid, the buildup of it in your body can create anxiety. There are herbal supplements like ashwagandha root and l-theanine (which is an amino acid that acts as a natural Prozac). Both of those will help with cortisol levels.

Supplements may not make the anxiety go away, but it can certainly remove one factor, or help support your body in one other way that it needed but wasn't receiving.

If you struggle with anxiety, I urge you to see your medical practitioner and talk to them. Find a professional counselor or a support group that can provide the backup you need. One of the best ways to nourish our soul is to find others that can understand our struggle.

When it comes to ANTS (automatic negative thoughts syndrome), you want to be prepared, but you also don't want to manifest the bad things by constantly thinking about them. Keep in mind that what you think is where you go. You have to be conscious and responsible, but if your brain keeps looping, and you can't seem to stop it, identifying why that's happening and taking steps to prevent it will help.

CHAPTER THIRTEEN

NOURISHING HABIT #11: EXERCISE

Exercise is an important part of health—whether we're talking about physical health or the health of the soul. But it's often an overstated challenge. A lot of my clients come to me after pushing their body so hard that it starts falling apart, or they're tired, or performance is lacking. We don't need to exercise to the point of exhaustion! That doesn't nourish our body or our soul.

In fact, we can get all the exercise we need in thirty minutes—even if we break that down into ten-minute increments throughout the day. Exercise is different for everyone. Do what you love. Work to put a habit in place that you can enjoy over the long haul.

Now *that's* my kind of workout!

Types of Exercise

There are countless ways to exercise, but a few of them that I always recommend to my clients are gentle walking (which is a really good starting point), weight lifting, and high-intensity interval training (HIIT). Gentle walking is a great place to start, then adding weights on top of it to get the additional benefits. When it comes to working out, keep in mind that doing a lot of things, and switching it up, is beneficial to our bodies.

If you're feeling good, healthy, and not breaking yourself down through working out, then it's great to try a little of everything. Walking, hiking, and weight lifting, for example, are supportive of all areas of your body. It can challenge you (like a hike), relax you (while on a walk), or help you build greater muscle and bone strength through weight training.

This also allows for the occasional day when you just aren't feeling like one particular exercise, or room to let your schedule breathe a little bit.

If you suspect that you have adrenal fatigue (which is something your naturopathic doctor can help you determine), then don't push yourself too much. Focus on the healing process, and more challenging exercise days can come later.

High-intensity interval training (HIIT) is an option when your body is healed and ready for a challenge. HIIT is doing more intense exercise for a shorter amount of time and then taking a rest (which creates the intervals). For example, you could do 45 seconds of jumping jacks, and then take 15 seconds to rest before doing it again. HIIT isn't restricted—you can do it for almost anything, such as:

1. Push-ups
2. Sit-ups
3. Sprints
4. Jumping Jacks
5. Squats

Here are a few other ideas for exercise to try out at whatever intensity feels good to you and does no harm.

1. Walking
2. Hiking
3. Walking hills
4. Light jogging
5. Sprints
6. Swimming
7. Pilates
8. Biking
9. Yoga
10. Tai Chi

Breaking Down Begets Building

Your body is in one of two states at any given moment: it's either building itself up or breaking down. When we push ourselves and work out hard, that breaks our body down. Breaking down isn't a bad thing as long as we move out of the breakdown phase and into the building phase. Breaking down helps us build our body back up later. Unfortunately, not enough of us move into the building up phase.

When we rest and give our body good food, that's the building phase. If we eat bad foods and miss sleep, we move our body to the breakdown phase. Exercising too much and not allowing ourselves time to recover makes it worse.

So how do we build ourselves back up?

By getting enough sleep and eating correctly. That allows us to really take care of ourselves and enable the body's natural building process to begin. We're constantly getting messages that something is broken in our body. When those come up, we need to listen. We can assist our body to build itself back up by treating the root problem and not the symptoms.

For example, heartburn is the body saying, "I'm on fire."

Heartburn isn't normal! Instead of popping a pill, a better starting point is trying a teaspoon of apple cider vinegar, drinking lemon water, or decreasing processed food. Then we're treating the cause, not the symptom.

A woman in her late seventies named Carmen came to see me to lose weight. While working through our initial visit, she confessed she had bad heartburn.

"I don't like to cook," she said. She often ate hot dogs for dinner. She would drink alcohol every single night. When she first started working with me, she began cutting back and making better choices. When she had a plateau, the only thing to do was to cut out alcohol completely. She did it for thirty days and got rid of her heartburn and walked all her boxes of medication over to her neighbor because she no longer needed it.

Like with heartburn, when the body gives us a sign about what is and isn't working, it's time to listen. Unless we deal with the things that are tearing us down, we won't heal in the long run, nor figure out our full capacity with our healthiest body.

I've seen firsthand through my own life, and my clients' lives, what stress does to our bodies.

When Jack and I started the divorce, sleep and relaxation were hard to come by. At this time, I was also going back to school, purchasing a home (which scared me half to death), and raising our kids. These were stressful times . . . sometimes sad and lonely times too.

Because of the stress and interrupted sleep, I started to get a band of belly fat around my midsection. I used food as comfort. To start building my body back up again, I initiated many nourishing habits, like going on walks, going to bed at a decent time, and cutting out alcohol.

After three days of the nourishing habits, I began to feel better. My sleep improved. My daily walks helped me clear my head. It was around this time that I realized that I would get depressed the day after I would have wine with my friends. After multiple times, I realized the correlation and decided to give wine up for a while.

Thanks to these habits, my body stopped breaking down. I could turn my focus back to nourishing my soul and being present for my family in a difficult time.

Instead of working yourself to the bone, trying to be faster, stronger, and better, and then getting frustrated when you're tired, hungry, or aren't losing weight, let's back up a step. Remember my guidance to *know yourself?* Here's a great place to do it.

Let's start by asking yourself a few questions:

1. Why are you working out so hard?

2. Are you trying to prove something?

3. Is it *really* serving you well?

Or maybe you're on the opposite spectrum. Instead of exercising too much, maybe you don't exercise at all. For you, I have the same path.

Answer these questions below:

1. Why aren't you exercising?

2. Are you avoiding something?

3. Is it serving you well?

A lot of my clients think that to lose weight, they have to suffer through extreme workouts, or just suffer in general. Whether that's through the physical pain of working out or major food deprivation, it doesn't feel *right* if they're not suffering.

Suffering is not a requirement!

Lifting weights helps you burn more calories and prevent your metabolism from slowing down, which is a common side effect of losing weight. But you don't have to be a professional weight lifter to get those results, nor do you have to run marathons either. Lifting weights is an easy way to increase your effectiveness without adding a lot of intensity.

The more muscle we have on our bodies, the more fat our bodies burn at a resting rate. You can burn more calories while watching Netflix! Just make sure you're losing weight in a supportive way instead of a painful way. If what you are doing supports and nurtures your body, you'll heal and keep the weight off. If it's done in a painful way, you won't keep the weight off.

Supportive is key.

The Benefits of Exercise

While we are walking and hitting our feet to the ground, we are actually building bone. Blood circulates. Our body fights stress. The effects and benefits of exercise go into the way we nourish our soul: exercise is proven to increase the production of serotonin (our happy hormone).[56]

Ashley was a college student who came to work with me in my office. My first impression was that she seemed so tired. Her shoulders slumped slightly. She had a glazed appearance every now and then and yawned during our discussion. When we started talking, her story came out.

"I've gained weight at college," she said. "It doesn't make sense! I do spin five days a week in the afternoon, which helps me wake up a little when my energy starts to dip. After all my classes, I just don't have the energy to get through the day. Sometimes working out helps. I just say to myself, *don't be lazy!* And then grab some more coffee."

Her comments had my mind instantly spinning. Unfortunately, this isn't an unusual case.

"When your energy is low," I said, "that's a signal. It doesn't mean that you need caffeine—you need rest and nutrients. Maybe even water. Although it seems counterintuitive, if you can get yourself to *rest* when you feel tired, you'll actually have more energy to work out later. It's not a matter of breaking down. It's building up."

Ashley learned that day how to do her own checklist and *know herself*. She asked herself the questions: *Why am I working out so hard? What do I need to prove? Do I feel any better?* We discussed working out in the morning, when her energy was high, and then allowing herself recovery time. In pushing through her workout and having coffee, she also impacted her sleep. Lessening her sleep only made the cycle worse.

Don't trip; just tie your laces. In other words, take time to stop and take care of the problem instead of just powering through.

Getting Started

Don't overthink exercise. Just take it one step at a time.

Joining a gym, signing up for new fitness classes, or making a workout date with friends can be helpful. Invest in small home weights, a mat, and a medicine ball. There are several reliable fitness and weight loss apps that can be very helpful as well.

CHAPTER FOURTEEN

NOURISHING HABIT #12: LIMIT YOUR STRESS

Don't skip this section if you think you aren't stressed. You might be surprised.

Some clients will swear to me that they aren't stressed. They feel fine, their life is good, and they wouldn't change a thing. But when I force them to look objectively at their life and possible stressors, they often realize they *are* stressed. They just didn't realize it.

Not surprisingly, this is typically the biggest challenge in creating nourishing habits. Stress increases hormones like adrenaline and cortisol, which is not something we want! Cortisol is a hormone that's produced in response to stress and causes the breakdown of muscle and fat storage in the abdominal area.[57]

When I have clients that have a really hard time losing weight, it's usually due to stress and cortisol. Long-term exposure to high cortisol and stress can be detrimental. Not fixing the source of stress can eventually exacerbate thyroid problems.

Increasing stress leads to a craving for carbs and sweets as well. It can lead to overeating and constant hunger. Eating more bread and sugar causes higher cravings and no satisfaction, which just perpetuates other cycles in our body that are equally unhealthy.

There's a cause-and-effect relationship with stress that most people don't intuitively know is there. It's not normal for things to start breaking in our body, even though we may think it is. Unfortunately, we're not always aware that we're constantly breaking down our body. We can only get away with that for so long.

One of the most important steps to decreasing stress is to be aware of it and then make changes. Here are a few ways to know if you're stressed and aren't aware:

1. You require coffee to start your day.
2. You feel like you just have to *push through* whatever it is you're going through.
3. At the end of the day, you relax with wine or alcohol in order to wind down.
4. When it's time to go to bed, you can't relax enough to sleep or have a hard time getting up in the morning.

When living in a stressful place, it's a problem of the parasympathetic brain versus the sympathetic brain. The sympathetic brain is our *fight or flight* response. It's keeping our body constantly geared to fight for our lives. When we face any kind of potential danger or challenge, the sympathetic brain activates. We aren't facing sabretooth tigers constantly anymore to need that backup, but of course, our body doesn't know that.

Some stress is inevitable. You can't run away from stress forever. The goal for creating a nourishing habit for your soul is to find a place of balance. When we put stress on our systems through exercise, for example, that can be normal. We just need to make sure we repair our systems by eating correctly and getting enough sleep afterward. That stimulates rebuilding.

The not-so-good-news is that as we age, we lose the ability to rebuild our body effectively. We still rebuild, just not as quickly. At that point, we need to be very careful about how much we allow ourselves to break down. Many of our day-to-day habits determine whether you're breaking down or building up, so paying careful attention to what we do every day can prevent this cycle.

Adrenal Fatigue

Adrenal fatigue happens when you have chronic lifestyle stress. You're constantly breaking down the body and living in a stressed-out state over a long period of time. This looks like the accumulation of drinking a lot of coffee, skipping meals, burning the candle at both ends, etc. People who struggle with this often describe themselves as *wired and tired*. They're constantly exhausted no matter what they do. This can happen to men and women equally.

When you're wired and tired, it means you're tired in the afternoon, but wired at night and not able to relax and sleep. You'll work all day, make dinner, relax, but then all of a sudden get wired again instead of going to bed. Eventually, you may stumble into bed at midnight and wake up early to start your day. Unfortunately, that's not enough time for our body to repair. Of course, you can be stressed without adrenal fatigue, so I always suggest that if you think this is a problem, find a naturopathic doctor to work with.

Adrenal fatigue is a tricky topic. Most western doctors don't recognize it exists, although you'll find integrative medicine doctors and naturopaths that can help you with it. Treating adrenal fatigue goes hand-in-hand with sleep. Your adrenal glands get taxed from constant stress and need a break. If they don't get it, eventually you'll start to see thyroid problems, which is another sign that there's a chronic stress problem.

Gray Hair

Not only does stress impact most of our body systems, but it can even change our hair color. A type of stress called *oxidative stress* happens in our body when free radicals (from pollution, poor diet, stress, etc.) outnumber our antioxidant defenses. Antioxidants usually come from a healthy diet.

Graying hair may be an indicator of oxidative stress-induced damage. Research has also shown that people with premature graying had a higher level of pro-oxidants and lower levels of antioxidants than those with normal hair.[58]

On top of all that, a vitamin B12 deficiency has also been linked to premature gray hair. There is at least one report of pigmentation returning to hair after the vitamin deficiency was resolved.[59]

This is exciting! It means that by lowering our stress and eating more antioxidants, we may have more control over whether our hair turns gray early on!

Why So Stressed?

If you're reading this section and seeing yourself in it (which could be almost all of us!) let's step back to my initial advice to *know yourself* and question everything. When we bring awareness to *why* you think you need those stressful things, it allows us to change. This is where we start questioning and go to the *why*, like we talked about earlier.

- Why are you drinking coffee?

  ....

  ....

- Why are you drinking wine?

  ....

  ....

- Why do you think you *need* it?

  ....

  ....

- What would happen if you stopped?

  ....

Think about it like this: why do people want alcohol at the end of the day? Why do so many people smoke? Their answers usually have to do with unwinding and removing the stress of the day. People think it helps, but both are actually toxic and not helpful! Some people smoke because it makes them stop and breathe. (Not that I want you to breathe in all those toxic chemicals!) Their goal is to relax their body.

To combat stress, I want you to breathe more, reduce or eliminate caffeine intake, and get more rest. I know that's hard. You're busy running a home, creating a career, living your life, and investing time in key people. It's well-established that interactions with pets and therapy animals can decrease stress in humans by decreasing cortisol levels and increasing oxytocin (the stress-relieving hormone). This is the same hormone that bonds mothers to their babies!

Here are a few other ideas to help you break the stress cycle:

1. Listen to a podcast.
2. Watch, read, or do something that will make you laugh.
3. Go for a walk.
4. Take a bath.
5. Write in your journal.
6. Call a best friend.
7. Meditate/Pray every day.
8. Consume more antioxidants.
9. Do some yoga.
10. Breathe deep.
11. Self-care is one of the surest ways to limit your stress.

CHAPTER FIFTEEN

NOURISHING HABIT #13: CELEBRATE YOUR WINS

Celebrate Your Wins

As part of every office visit or every call I have with my clients, we start off by discussing a win.

I define a win as something that went well in the last week. No matter how difficult the week was, there is always something we can find (sometimes we have to look it over together) that was a win.

For example, when I was trying to get off sugar years ago, I had a hard time. While struggling, I decided to go to the lesser of evils. Instead of turning to bread when I had a craving, I went to trail mix. It still got me a step away from the thing I was really addicted to, and added more protein and fat, which was a win. Then I celebrated that decision. It got me away from feeling like a failure for not being perfect.

Wins for my clients are varied, but here are a few examples that I love:

- I only ate one cookie instead of seven!
- I met my goal of tracking all my meals.

- I went on a ten-minute walk.
- I drank up to my goal in water.
- I didn't drink any soda this week.
- I went to a basketball game and didn't eat junk food.
- Instead of saying to myself, "I'm a failure," I said, "I now have more information for next time this happens. I haven't failed."

Celebrating our wins is so important! Not only does it give us a more positive outlook on what the past week has been like, but it gives us an opportunity to express gratitude. Maybe it would have been better for me to have nothing at all instead of the trail mix. Am I going to beat myself up for the chocolate chips in the trail mix? No. Because I did better than yesterday, and I can be grateful for that.

When we focus on the things that went right instead of the things that went wrong, we are more likely to succeed. In fact, one study has shown[60] that maintaining a positive outlook in times of stress can decrease inflammation and later depression. Gratitude literally prevents us from getting depressed in difficult times.

Plus, it gets easier as it goes. My clients end up paying attention to their wins outside our calls and telling me about them as soon as our call starts!

When we get to a point where we can be thankful for the things we have (and are not totally focused on what we don't have), we've arrived at a good place. What better method for nourishing the soul can there be?

Be Your Own Cheerleader

My clients often tell me, "Julie, I heard your voice in my head when I stared down that sugary donut, or eyed that glass of wine after a long day. Or when I changed one habit, you said to me in my head, 'You're doing great!'" That *is* great, but what's even better is when they start hearing their own positive voice. I call it the inner cheerleader.

There are a lot of gurus out there to help cheer you on, but in the end, *you* should be your own biggest cheerleader to make it past the finish line.

In order to succeed, we have to have tools in our toolbox that get us to our healthiest body, and one of those is the ability to cheer ourselves on. We have to go through hard things to get to the other side and to become stronger. The more we believe in ourselves along the way, the better. You have to be your own cheerleader.

This goes deeper than just rooting yourself to your goals. Even if everyone else thinks you're the smartest person or the top producer or the best mom, what does it mean if you don't believe them? You have to allow yourself to believe them. You have to start telling yourself it's true. This takes time. It's something you have to build upon (which is why this is a nourishing habit that you get into every day). It can feel foreign. Maybe it *is* foreign if you never had a cheerleader. Even if you had the best parents and most supportive family, you'll still need to give this gift to yourself. I grew up feeling loved and cared for, but eventually realized that in life I would have to learn how to cheer myself on. If you're not used to it, you learn it over time. It's a skill.

Working with my clients has helped me see that a lot of people just avoid stuff. Instead of dealing with their problem, knowing themselves, or finding support, they eat, run, or drink alcohol. Learning how to cheer yourself on can get you through the things we'd rather avoid. Those who cheer themselves on tend to have greater success and better health.

CHAPTER SIXTEEN

NOURISHING HABIT #14: GIVE YOURSELF GRACE

One of the most important nourishing habits you can learn from this book is to give yourself grace. When we're wrapped up in our own lives, we don't always see how good we're doing. Because we juggle everything on a daily basis, we forget how much it can be.

I am blessed to be the outside perspective that can remind women of how good they are doing. Sometimes, that's hard to remember, because it can seem like we're constantly on the path of what we want to do, and then things come up to derail us.

Although this is the last of the nourishing habits I'm setting out, it may be one of the most important. The relentless pursuit of perfection means a lot of my clients fail, which is normal, and then get upset. We end up sabotaging ourselves. Giving ourselves grace is the power that can help us overcome whatever stands in our way.

Giving yourself grace is kind of like becoming your own cheerleader. It helps us cheer ourselves on and live our best lives. Really, giving yourself grace is giving yourself permission. Permission to be imperfect. Permission to try again. Permission to fail.

Where would we be without that?

Consistency

The best plan you can be on is the consistent one. When the tough times come, remember that the best thing you can do is get back to those nourishing habits. Be consistent in one or two things—they can act as alternatives.

Also, consider this question if you're being hard on yourself. What's your alternative to the nourishing habit? You certainly could go back to what you were doing before. Whether that's snacking like crazy, eating at 3:00 in the morning, sleeping four hours a night, or laying on the couch instead of going for a walk. You could go back there and do those things again. But why? This is another great place for you to know yourself.

Give yourself grace for the weeks that come up and are harder than others. You fell off? Okay. Now get back on. It's normal to fall off. It's *better* to get back on. It's normal to veer away for a moment and need to come back. So come back. Start at one nourishing habit, then add another one back the next day. Did you binge wine last night? Keep to your fast today. Eat a balanced breakfast. Tell yourself, "That wasn't a failure, only feedback." Then find the feedback.

Even if you aren't perfect, getting back to the habits helps you stay consistent. You don't go as far down the next shiny squirrel path. Consistency, notice, doesn't mean *perfection*.

One of my clients, Shannon, came to one of our appointments and said, with panic in her voice, "I went out with my girlfriends this weekend and decided to have just one glass of wine. I stuck to that, but then I ate an entire cheese platter!"

"That's okay," I said. "Just get right back on track the next day.

You are human, and things happen. Don't beat yourself up. It's time to give yourself some grace and come back to the consistent path. Wine brings your inhibitions down, and you get pulled around. Now come back to consistency."

It may feel awkward at first. You may say, "Why even try again?" The answer is this: because you're worth it. You didn't fail.

Better health is one step away.

Shiny Squirrel Syndrome

Most people see the shiny paths that take them away from their goal and chase them relentlessly. We're like puppies that see a squirrel and get pulled away in an instant, forgetting all our hard work or previous focus. That's actually normal.

If it happens to you, it's okay. It's time to give yourself grace for those moments when you do fall prey to the shiny squirrel. Step back. Have a moment of gratitude. Celebrate one win for the day. Write in your journal. Go for a walk. These sound familiar, right? The beauty of the nourishing habits is the tapestry they create when they weave through our lives. Overall, one thread at a time, we get stronger and stronger. Giving ourselves the grace to fail, start again, and keep going is the key.

You're doing a lot. You can only do the things you can do. Sometimes, that needs to be enough.

When my clients have a down week—or a bad week where they fell prey to shiny squirrel syndrome—I end up giving them a pep talk. Most of the time, it's a reminder.

"You've had a little disappointment," I'll say. "But you're still on the path. You haven't knocked yourself off because you saw the shiny squirrel. You're still here. You're in it. Let's keep going and keep that ultimate *why* in mind."

I'm saying that right now to you, too.

Change always requires mental work. When you're learning to live in a way that naturally supports what you need, you may encounter mental challenges as well as physical. Our goal in nourishing our body is to achieve a balance where we feel good, have energy, and can live the life we want.

Something that I see underrepresented in the search for energy and happiness is the power of our habits to determine our outcomes. Now that we've come to the end of establishing the science behind our habits, Part Four is going to walk you through the steps of creating your own nourishing habits, one at a time, so you can be successful.

PART FOUR

START YOUR
Nourishing
HABITS

CHAPTER SEVENTEEN

MINDSET

At the beginning of the book, we briefly spoke about the importance of mindset in helping you find your healthiest body. The way you talk to yourself, knowing yourself, and looking at your habits, are all part of that. Now we're going to dive a little deeper.

I'm willing to say that better health is all mindset. You can't change your mindset until you're aware of your habits. If you don't have the proper mindset, it's not going to work.

So, how do you go about changing your mindset? I have four easy steps that we'll review right here, then dive into deeper.

1. **Awareness.** Cultivate awareness by looking at your body or paying attention to how it feels. What signals is it giving you? Are you tired? Restless? Edgy? Learn what's going on. What's working? What isn't working? Choose one thing you want to work on, whether it's a thought or a habit.

2. **Change your habits.** Tell yourself that you *can* do this. You are worth the change. Things will work this time. Give yourself permission to succeed through consistency and planning.

3. **New habits.** Replace your old habit (or thought) with new ones. Trying to eat healthier? When you reach for the chips, grab some pickles instead. When you are certain you have to have caffeine, drink a glass of water, or take a nap.

4. **Patience.** Allow this to take some time. Up to sixty-six days, but it may occur sooner for some, or longer for others. Older habits die hard, so you may need to really stick with it!

Awareness

We first have to be aware of what we're doing—and what our body is telling us—before we can make the next best decision. Nourishing yourself requires a mindset shift in four different ways:

1. Paying attention to your current thoughts and habits.
2. Becoming aware of what you do.
3. Becoming aware of why you do it.
4. Changing based on your new awareness.

Most people aren't aware of the state their body is in. Are you tired, bloated, filled with anxiety, or depressed? Or is it that you just have a little weight to lose? Whatever state your body is in, the first step is being aware.

With awareness comes the need to get clear on *why* you want this change. Let's take getting healthy, for example. What will better health do for you? What will it give you? How will your life change from better health?

So many of my clients come into my office and say, "I wasn't aware my body was so stressed," or "I had no idea that I snacked so much!" Once we become aware, we can make changes from the right information. What is getting in our way?

Oftentimes . . . it's us.

"Deciding to commit yourself to long-term results rather than short-term fixes is as important as any decision you'll make in your lifetime."
–Tony Robbins

In order to truly change—and make it lasting—we need to come up with a plan based on awareness of who we are and what we're currently facing. Can you imagine what we can accomplish with the power of our nourishing habits behind us?

Anything.

Awareness creates a place of safety from which to act. When willpower and motivation totally fail us, nourishing habits keep us aware of what we need to be successful. It also cultivates change. You can only change bad habits when you know they're there. As a general rule, we tend to make things harder than they need to be. Becoming aware of yourself, your body, and your current habits is the first true step to your best health and most powerful life.

I tell my clients to look for the light bulb moment. That's when the light bulb turns on in your mind, and you suddenly understand, it helps us see that we're successful and why we *haven't* been successful in the past. There has to be that *click*. That moment of, "Oh, okay! I get it! I can do it." It's when you have the feeling that you've gathered all the information and can now proceed.

You might realize *I've been skipping lunch every day. Then I'm totally starving and craving chocolate later in the day.* From there, you can make sure to eat lunch and beat those cravings before they come.

Kim is super busy as an outside sales representative. When she heard how great intermittent fasting was, she began to fast by skipping breakfast, but she still drank a pot of coffee. She ate a healthy salad around lunch and then didn't eat again until 6:00 p.m. At 9:30 p.m., she was starving overnight. She wasn't losing any weight and came to me in tears and frustration.

"Stop eating three hours before bed, and go back to a more moderate twelve-hour fast," I told her. "Eat every three hours during the day and only consume only one cup of coffee."

The coffee was causing too much cortisol in her body and giving her a false sense of being full. With drinking that, she never had time or room to drink her water. After implementing my suggestions, she had better sleep, better success, and wasn't so hungry at the end of the day.

That is what awareness and living with your nourishing habits looks like.

Change Habits

After we find more awareness, we then have a unique opportunity to change. Some habits may be so old that we aren't even sure how they got there! Let's start with the following questions to see if you have old habits that could use some revamping:

1. What habits have you put in place and why?

_____

_____

2. Can you bring greater awareness to things that need work by simply *looking* at them?

_____

_____

3. What isn't working right now?

_____

....

I often tell my clients, "It's hard for us to change, but it's easy to change our habits."

Are you saying to yourself, _Julie, are you crazy? It's not easy to change my habits!_ Time to go back to the questions in the previous section and find out why you think that way. What you may find is that part of the limiting belief of _it's too hard_ is because we operate from our old experiences.

Our inner person can only operate from what we know. When, for example, you're given an opportunity or asked to do something outside of your comfort zone (which is established from previous experiences), you'll probably feel fearful and uncertain. It's outside of the familiar. That's totally normal. We just don't want to stop there.

Let's say you're going to the grocery store and your habit has you reaching for a bag of potato chips. Can you set the chips down and steer your cart to the produce aisle? You can. Since you've already put in these habits, you just switch up the details. Change the groceries you buy, the way you exercise, or how you prepare your dinners. Instead of potato chips, reach for apples.

Habits can take up to sixty-six days to develop,[61] which means we need to invest in repetition. I love the rubber band analogy. A loose rubber band is like our regular life. Easy, loose, not too difficult. But when we pull it, we're changing our normal state. We need to pull that band for sixty-six days for the change to stick so we don't bounce back to what we did before.

Jessica signed up to work with me for twelve weeks. From the beginning, she seemed to go into a panic with every interaction we had. Instead of talking with me for an hour, reviewing her questions, discussing her best path, and discussing what she'd learned, she would text me and say, *I don't want to discuss all of this on the phone with you. Texting only.*

When I tried to talk to her about meal prepping on the weekends, she had an immediate excuse. *That's my family time,* she said in a text. Broaching the idea of using an app or a journal to track what she ate (and bring more awareness to her habits) also met with immediate resistance.

She had a deep fear of change that she didn't want to work through, which made it impossible to improve her life. She wanted to keep her old habits and try to be accountable to me. As a result, she had no progress.

New Habits

Once you've cultivated awareness and decided on a plan for changing that habit, it's time to move into the new habit.

My clients often struggle with their new habits simply because of what they're telling themselves. If you always tell yourself that something (like getting healthier, losing weight, or lowering your cholesterol) is too hard, it will be too hard. It will seem like work.

Are you telling yourself that a new habit is too difficult? Are you telling yourself that you *aren't* something *(I'm not strong enough; I'm not good enough; I'm not perfect enough.)*? Sometimes you have to just stop, clear your mind, and let yourself hear your thoughts. They can spin in the background of our minds without us even knowing it.

We tend to make things harder than we need to by thinking we can't change, or our habits are set and won't move. All of this begs the question, *what can we change?* How do we get rid of these beliefs? If you think that living with nourishing habits is going to be too difficult, let's change that by exploring this a little deeper.

Here comes that mindset work!

Think of the problem that you're telling yourself is too hard. Now ask yourself these questions:

1. Is it actually hard? (Or does it just *seem* hard?)
2. Did I have an experience in the past that I'm allowing to dictate what will happen now?
3. Can it be easy?

While working with one client we'll call Janice, I was often surprised by how often she said, "This is just too hard. I can't do this."

Peeling back the layers revealed a busy woman with a career, active children, a beautiful, organized house, and only twenty pounds to lose. She ran around all day doing everything for everybody else except for herself. When we began working together, she truly wasn't aware of how much she wasn't taking care of herself.

Her usual refrain would sometimes appear up to twenty times in our hour-long call. "It's too hard for me, Julie. It's just too hard for me."

"Janice," I said one day, "are you aware of how much you say, *'it's too hard'*?"

"Really?"

"You've said it at least twenty times now in this session alone."

She paused. "Oh," she said. "I didn't realize."

"Can other people do this? Is it too hard for them?"

She thought about it and said, "No. Other people can do it."

"Can you?"

"Yes. I can."

She hadn't even *realized* she was saying that it was too hard for her to do—it was like she went on autopilot. She had no awareness! She didn't truly want to do the work right then, so it seemed like a lot of work. With that burden on her, she never would have committed to her goal and started into a new habit.

Another example I've seen of this mindset problem was with Anna. After attending the Phillies training camp in Florida with her son, she came back, set her purse on the table in my office, and declared, "Oh my God. It's impossible to eat healthy on the road!"

Further exploration revealed that she had stopped at a few fast food restaurants and was now battling renewed cravings for them again.

"Is it totally impossible to eat healthy on the road," I asked, "or does it just seem that way? Would other people be able to eat healthy while traveling?"

Anna stopped and thought. "Well . . . yes."

Of course, it *isn't* impossible to eat healthy while traveling, but she had a mindset, no awareness of it, and no new habit created to replace the old one. This caused her to eat unhealthily, renew her cravings, and white knuckle it through those cravings until they had subsided again.

This is where we make it harder on ourselves than it needs to be. By cultivating awareness of our mind and our body, and killing our cravings, we can get rid of their power over us entirely. That, in turn, leads to greater health.

At the end of our conversation, Anna said, "Oh, I see it now. It's actually just easiest to eat out, but not impossible to eat healthy."

These thoughts—and our lack of awareness—give us permission

to fail. So what does permission to succeed look like? It looks like consistency. Like not giving up, establishing nourishing habits, then consistently staying with them. We put things into place to protect us so that it's easier for us to take care of ourselves and slay our goals.

In the next chapter, we're going to start creating your own habits.

We're going to create accountability in this process by making sure you write down the habits that you're putting into place. But it's not enough to just write them down. Put them somewhere so you can see them all the time, whether that's on your phone, written on your bathroom mirror, or on your refrigerator.

Keep in mind as you go through this process that health isn't one-size-fits-all. What works for you right now may not be needed later—that's fine. You can always revisit this book, go back through the process, and figure out what you need at your current stage in life. A young mom with several kids will have different needs than a woman going through menopause.

Besides, as you create awareness and form new habits, you'll change. Your mindset will improve and shift, which is just what we want! You can always come back, figure out what nourishing habit you need next, and keep moving forward. Just like in our business, we tackle one challenge, then the next!

We owe it to ourselves and to the world to be the best version of ourselves.

Patience

The final step in managing your mindset and allowing successful change revolves around giving yourself grace. Have patience with the process. You'll fall off the bandwagon, but that's okay. Be patient with yourself. Climb back on.

There's a false belief circulating around out there that says *willpower is enough*. Willpower is a little bit of a myth that I'd like to debunk. Willpower often fades, which is why I work with so many clients. They look to me for accountability or a support system at the moment their willpower wavers. Most people just need a safety net!

This doesn't mean that we have failed if our willpower fades—it's just part of the busy lives we lead. You almost always have enough willpower to start a new thing, whether that's a diet, a lifestyle change, a new way of eating, or a new exercise routine. Then life happens. Troubles pop up. Plateaus happen. Kids get sick. All of these factors erode our willpower, which often fades away. Even though you may start out with enough willpower to start a healthier lifestyle, it may wear down eventually. You'll come face-to-face with one of your triggers, and your willpower may not be there to save you.

Your nourishing habits will. Motivation fades, consistent habits don't.

Selena's seven-month-daughter was hospitalized for difficulty breathing less than two months after Selena and I began to work together. Up to that point, Selena had been successful with cleaning up her eating habits, fasting at night, and drinking more water.

"I'm feeling really good," she said during our phone call. "My daughter is stable, and I'm able to order clean foods while we're here. So far, I'm a little more stressed, but it's okay. In fact, it's a little bit easier because I'm solely focused on my daughter, and don't have to worry about stuff at home."

Her daughter remained in the hospital for a week before going home. We kept up over text messages. Then, after things settled down, we hopped on the phone for another call. Despite her previous strength while under stress in the hospital, things had changed.

"It's like all my willpower faded the moment I knew we were coming home," Selena said. "We left the hospital and immediately had to coordinate with the home oxygen company. I could suddenly feel my exhaustion from the lack of sleep. My in-laws had been watching my son, and they had other family members over when we returned, leading to a very full, loud house. As soon as I walked in the door, my dogs were barking because they needed a walk. The home oxygen company called. My daughter cried. My son suddenly needed all my attention, not to mention the emails and work I'd missed the last week. In all this chaos, we were trying to manage a young infant with oxygen and a major lack of sleep.

"Then I looked at the counter and saw that my mother-in-law had made a batch of her famous cookies. All the previous willpower I had at the hospital disappeared. I had one, then two, and suddenly I had downed five."

So what happens when our willpower fades, like Selena?

How do we recover?

We put the healthy habits back into place and give ourselves grace. My philosophy has always been around the 80/20 rule. Eating healthy 80% of the time and enjoying those not so healthy foods and drinks 20% of the time. It's about moderation, not deprivation.

To Selena, I said, "It's okay. You've been through a lot and were so strong. Now it's time to remember your nourishing habits. Don't let frustration over the cookies make it worse. Get back into those habits now."

Selena and I spoke at length about her situation after she reported what happened. I reminded her of her goal, helped her give herself a little grace because of all she'd been through, and helped nudge her back toward taking care of herself.

All of us face situations like Selena's. Nourishing habits are there to catch us when the willpower fades, and we feel as if we've stumbled. Keep in mind that the nourishing habits are there to protect you, but that doesn't mean you have to be perfect.

Feedback, Not Failure

This is the perfect time to remind you that *there is no failure, only feedback.*

No one is perfect, and that's okay. When an inevitable slip off the bandwagon happens, say to yourself, "There is no failure, only feedback." Not only will this keep you from spiraling even worse, but it's a powerful way to practice positive self-talk.

Maybe you slide away from your new nourishing habit for a day or two. Before you slide into a dark place where you think of your failure, remember that this is data. It's not failure. You only fail if you stop showing up and stop trying.

For example, let's say that you started having gratitude every day. As part of that, you write five things in your journal every day in the morning. But a sick kiddo, an unexpected visitor, work appointments, or summer vacation gets in the way. Four days pass before you realize you've not once recorded your gratitude. This is when it's time to step back and say, "This isn't failure. This is only feedback."

The feedback is that you didn't sleep well the night before, or you overcommitted yourself, or got sick, or got into a fight with your spouse, or your kids came home from school brokenhearted, and you forgot to be grateful.

How can you alter when those circumstances come up? Can you plan ahead next time?

Like Selena, you take the feedback, make a plan, and keep going.

The 80/20 Rule

Sometimes we think we have to be perfect.

After years of working with clients, I can confidently say that if you do your best and keep tracking, good things will happen.

Jenni had a meltdown one day on a call with me because she didn't know what to eat. "There are bad oils at every restaurant," she said. "I don't want to eat anything cooked in unhealthy oils! Now I'm just not eating out."

I immediately sought to calm her. "No," I said, "it's okay. You just do your best. Do better than you did before. Instead of fries, get a vegetable. This isn't a question of perfection. This is just about doing everything you can."

You can't be 100% all the time, which is why I have the 80/20 rule. Stay firmly with your nourishing habits 80% of the time, and the 20% you aren't totally with them, you'll still be safe. When it comes to implementing this new lifestyle, don't get paralyzed by the *best* of everything. Don't stop eating because you can't get organic food for every single meal, or a friend cooked with an oil that isn't as healthy.

It will be okay. Remember to give yourself grace.

For example, let's say you used to eat bagels every morning for breakfast, but now you're eating eggs and doing much better. One day you're at a work conference, and all they have is food you wouldn't eat at home, including bagels and cream cheese. What do you do?

Look for nutrients, and do the best you can.

Maybe it's not what you would have expected to eat, but you did your best. What more can anyone ask? If you're expecting perfection, you'll set yourself up to fail.

If your first plan doesn't work, keep going. Just don't stop. Remember that permission to succeed looks like consistency. Start small, changing three things at first, and then add to them from there. Look at this as walking up a hill to your healthiest you! You don't have to be fast, but in time, the view from the top is breathtaking. If you fall off the wagon, climb back on right away. Don't beat yourself up. Don't wallow.

Just keep going.

You can do this.

CHAPTER EIGHTEEN

THE FOUR STEPS TO SUCCESS

Step One: Set Your Goal

The first place we start is figuring out your ultimate goal. What do you want to create safety around in your daily life so that you *know* it will happen?

At the beginning of the book, I had you write down your goals, your desires, your wishes for better health. It's time to revisit that. If you didn't list out your goals, do so now.

Here's the list of goals my clients often come to me with again:

1. Lose weight.
2. Sleep better.
3. Have healthier skin.
4. Heal my digestive tract.
5. Increase confidence.
6. Improve fitness.
7. Fix nutrition.
8. Better health.
9. More energy.
10. Prevent disease.

Setting your goal is going to help us establish the nourishing habits you need to start with. For this, I suggest you choose two goals: one for your body, one for your soul.

For example: if your goal is to lose thirty pounds, we'll have a greater emphasis on food accountability, fasting, and gentle exercise. If your goal is to do more self-care, we'll look more at the things that fill you with joy and how to get more of them into your schedule.

You can establish a goal that isn't directly related to one of the fourteen habits I've listed. But I suggest that you start with at least one of the nourishing habits from this book so you learn my process, and can then put it into place. From there, you can take this structure and make nourishing habits that may be more applicable or detailed for your situation. I'll provide space for you to fill in other habits that you want to create.

All habits are intertwined, and some are non-negotiable no matter what your goal. (Everyone needs self-care, for example.) But having your goal and keeping it top of mind also helps provide the initial motivation you need to change. Then, when motivation and willpower fails, you'll already have habits set into place that keep you from falling off the cliff.

Step Two:
Know What Works for You

Once you've decided what you want most (for now!), we want to figure out what already works best for you.

Let's say that your goal is to lower your blood pressure. The next best step is to figure out what isn't working for you now, and what does (or could possibly) work for you moving forward. Turn to your paper and draw a line down the middle. Write out two columns: **What Doesn't Work** and **What Does Work.** Fill those out based on your goal.

Here's an example below:

Goal: To lower my blood pressure.

What Doesn't Work	**What Does Work**
1. Eating really sugary foods.	1. Check-ins with my doctor.
2. Gaining weight.	2. Gentle exercise.
3. Watching TV instead of exercising.	3. Checking blood pressure regularly.
4. Really intense exercise.	4. Losing weight.
	5. Eating more fiber.
	6. Focus on consuming less sodium.

Figuring out what works for you is another way to cultivate awareness from the beginning. Although the options listed above may seem overly simple or obvious, sometimes it's not that obvious. Like my client that didn't even realize she kept saying, "It's too hard." Getting down to the base layer of what's in our mind can make us more successful.

Step Three:
Replace Old Habits with New Ones

Once we've worked through the first two steps, it becomes about replacing what you do with what you *want* to be doing. When we have bad habits, we need to replace them with better habits.

Think of it this way: you're already going into the kitchen to drink coffee and eat something after you wake up in the morning, so you just have to replace one habit with a healthier habit. Instead of drinking coffee, switch to drinking water. If you have to, buy a special water bottle, or even put it in your coffee cup if you're attached to that part of the ritual. Instead of pouring a bowl of sugary cereal, grab food full of nutrients. If every day at 5:00 p.m. you want wine, intentionally replace it with something else like tea, lemon water, or sparkling water with lemon.

No matter what you think is normal, the truth is that your body isn't craving coffee, wine, or chocolate. It's craving nourishment.

Step Four: Repetition

This is where the hard work comes into play.

Now that we know the new habit we need to form, we have to make it happen. Again and again and again. Remember, it takes around sixty-six days to form a habit, so we have to keep putting in the work. Keep reaching for water or tea instead of sugar.

Despite science showing us that it takes most people sixty-six days to create their new habit, it truly varies for everyone. Some of my clients that remove sugar from their diet report that within seven days the cravings are gone or have subsided. Others say it takes weeks. While they may not have made it a full *habit* yet, it becomes much easier nonetheless.

Before you decide on the nourishing habits you start, make sure to set yourself up for success. If you decide to tell people in your life about your goals and enlist their support, this can be a huge step. Not only will you have support from others, but you won't be doing it alone. When tempting or difficult circumstances arise, they can help you stay in check.

This is where the importance and power of positive self-talk becomes key, because the process can be frustrating. Remember—you are enough. You have the power to move mountains. Decide today that enough is enough. You will not feed your body bad things or toxins anymore.

You are too precious, and the world needs your gifts.

Now, let's work together in the next chapter to start implementing this process.

CHAPTER NINETEEN

START IMPLEMENTING YOUR NOURISHING HABITS

Now we're going to start creating your new habits—one at a time. The whole goal behind *Nourishing Your Body and Soul* is to keep this real-world focused. If you try to start too many habits at one time, you're going to get overwhelmed, and you won't be successful. If you focus on *only* nourishing your body, you may suffer in mindset, motivation, and focus. That's why I walk my clients through a step-by-step, weekly process toward their individual goals and personality. I also recommend that you focus on a habit that nourishes your body, and follow it with one that nourishes your soul.

In this next part, I'll take you through the fourteen nourishing habits we discussed through the book, then give you checkboxes to mark off when you've done it.

Seven days are provided for each habit for you to track and take notes about each new nourishing habit. These appear in alternating order—one habit for the body, one habit for the soul—so you can work through them one at a time. Or you can pick which one you start with and move through. Keep it to one habit at a time. Not only will that prevent overwhelm, but it will help you really focus, ask your body what it's feeling, and make this work for what you need.

You may not need seven days to start a new habit. You may already have these in place—if so, skip that week, or recommit to it at 100% to see if it changes anything. Getting away from what is good for us often happens slowly, in increments, and this can help pull you back. I've also provided blank habits for you to fill in on your own at the end of this section.

If it seems like too much to write it all down or keep up with it, do your best. Then try to do a little better the next day. Even if you *try* and don't see it through, the feedback will help you sculpt an even more tailored plan moving forward.

There are blank spaces available for you to write in your own answers or options as well.

PROTECT YOUR SLEEP

There is no denying that sleep is crucial to health for both body and soul. Everyone will have different sleep needs, which is why I have several ideas for establishing a better habit around bedtime.

Read through my suggestions below, and keep them in mind as you decide your best, new nourishing habit around sleep.

Ways to protect your sleep:

1. Keep your room on the cool side. Studies show that an important signal for sleep onset is lowering our core body temperature.[62]
2. Turn off EMF's (electromagnetic fields). These are on our computers and smartphones. They call out to our brain at night, interrupting our sleep.[63]
3. Light shuts off melatonin, which is the hormone that helps us sleep, so keep everything dark, and limit lights at night. Keep low light in the house in the evening, and use the night light feature on your phone.
4. Use dark out shades if you need to.
5. Take supplements, like magnesium, potassium, 5-HTP, Glycine, or L-theanine.
6. Set a goal to have eight or nine hours of uninterrupted sleep (if possible!). Then evaluate how you feel. Did your

day go better on nine hours? Or are you feeling rested with eight? Whatever feedback you get, go with that.

Pick one of the suggestions below, and implement it as a nourishing habit for the next seven days. Be sure to come back and write down how you feel, as well as any feedback that you gathered, in the space provided below.

Once you're done testing the new nourishing habit, there's space to make a new plan for the next week.

1. **Establish a sleep routine.** This is not only beneficial, but crucial to finding our healthiest state and recovering our energy. Our body loves routine, particularly when sleep is on the line. By establishing a routine, you can start training your body to wind down. Let's say you go to bed at 10:00 p.m. By 7:00 p.m., plan on getting your dishes done, putting on your jammies, turning your lights down, brushing your teeth, and switching to night mode on your phone. This doesn't mean you should rush to clean the house until 10:00, then play games on your phone from 10:00-10:30! You want your body to make melatonin and not get a second wind. Instead of winging it (and falling asleep on the couch until midnight), get into that consistent routine.

2. **Limit work or computer stuff at night.** I know how hard this is. Setting that boundary is difficult, but so worth it for long-term sleep management. Even if you love your work or watching Netflix, there will still be an element of stress if you participate in it right before bed. Read a book instead of being on your computer or smart phone. Turn

off your Wi-Fi if your phone is next to you so you aren't tempted.

3. **Avoid caffeine and chocolate.** Both are a stimulant and will keep you awake or disrupt sleep cycles, even if you had them earlier in the day. If you must have them, set a time, like 3:00 p.m., that way you won't eat them later in the day.

Working Through the New Habit Steps

1. **Step One: What initial change works for you?**
   a. Set an alarm on your phone for when it's time to start your pre-bedtime routine.
   b. Tell your family members your plan so they're on board with you.
   c. Get an app on your phone that limits blue light after 7:00.
   d. _____
   e. _____
   f. _____

2. **Step Two: Replace old habits.**

   a. What are your old habits?

   _____
   _____
   _____

   b. What will you replace them with?

   _____
   _____
   _____

c. How will this change positively benefit you?

_____

_____

_____

3. **Step Three: Over the next seven days, focus on your sleep routine.** If you notice any changes, don't be afraid to take notes in the space provided below. These can help you have added motivation later. Ask yourself the following questions as the week progresses:

a. How do I feel?

_____

_____

_____

b. What has changed?

_____

_____

_____

c. How does my body feel?

_____

_____

_____

GRATITUDE

We already know that gratitude has undeniable power, which is why I have all of my clients implement it shortly after we start working together. There are several ways to integrate gratitude into our daily lives. (It's one of the most powerful ways to feed your soul.)

Pick one of the suggestions below, and implement it as a nourishing habit for the next seven days. Be sure to come back and write down how you feel, as well as any feedback that you've gathered, in the space provided below. Once you're done testing the new nourishing habit, there's space to make a new plan for the next week.

1. **Don't take on problems.** In order to get to a better place of gratitude, make sure you aren't getting dumped on with people's problems. Allowing people to walk all over you will make it very difficult to be in a position of gratitude and positive thinking.
2. **Meditation.** Spend time thinking about what you're grateful for. Focus on little things, like having a roof over your head, food in the refrigerator, or gas in the car.
3. **Express your gratitude.** Being grateful *and* expressing that gratitude is a strong way to feel it. The positive aspects of gratitude are even better when we hear it out loud, and a

double benefit is others then hear it. It's also a powerful relationship connection.

Working Through the New Habit Steps

1. **Step One: What initial change works for you?**
   a. Write down 3-5 things you're grateful for.
   b. Do one act of service every day.
   c. Pick a new person every day, and tell them you're grateful for them.
   d. _____
   e. _____
   f. _____

2. **Step Two: Replace old habits.**

   a. What are your old habits?

   _____

   _____

   b. What will you replace them with?

   _____

   _____

   c. How will this change positively benefit you?

   _____

   _____

3. **Step Three: Over the next seven days, focus on gratitude.** If you notice any changes, don't be afraid to take notes in the space provided below. These can help you have added motivation later. Ask yourself the following questions as the week progresses:

a. How do I feel?

_____
_____
_____
_____

b. What has changed?

_____
_____
_____
_____

c. How does my body feel?

_____
_____
_____
_____

DRINKING LEMON WATER

When it comes to creating new habits, many of my clients begin with drinking warm lemon water in the morning. It's the perfect place to start! Not only will you feel better with more water, and have better health, but it's the easiest thing because you have water right there. Plus, everyone has to drink water (in some form) to survive.

When you start drinking warm water with lemon, I caution you to go slow at first. The warm water seems to enhance the taste, so you may want to start with a quarter of a lemon per day. Squeeze the juice in the warm water, or add it to some tea that has a complimentary taste. Over time, gradually increase to half a lemon.

Some of my clients will squeeze the lemon juice into the warm water, then let the piece of lemon sit in it for an extra boost. Just don't feel like you have to do this right away if it's too strong. Do it at whatever level will keep you motivated to do it and not feel like too much.

Pick one of the suggestions below, and implement it as a nourishing habit for the next seven days. Be sure to come back and write down how you feel, as well as any feedback that you've gathered, in the space provided below. Once you're done testing the new nourishing habit, there's space to make a new plan for the next week.

1. **Pick a favorite cup.** Even if you have to go buy one, having an item to attach a routine to can help us gain more success. Use that cup every morning for your warm water with lemon. If you have to, leave it sitting out by your sink so you see it.

2. **Create accountability.** Put a piece of paper up on your fridge with seven boxes. Check them off each day that you have the warm water with lemon. Visibility keeps the reminder fresh.

3. **Prepare for success.** Make sure you achieve this habit by implementing preparation. I love it when people prepare! Schedule the time on your calendar. Wake up before anyone else. Enjoy the time while you sip the warm water with lemon. Cut the wedges up beforehand. Buy enough lemons for the week.

Working Through the Steps

1. **Step One: What initial change works for you?**
   a. Telling a family member about your new goal.
   b. Drink the warm water with lemon from a special cup.
   c. Tracking it on an app.
   d. _____
   e. _____
   f. _____

2. **Step Two: Replace old habits.**

a. What are your old habits?

_____

_____

b. What will you replace them with?

_____

_____

c. How will this change positively benefit you?

_____

_____

3. **Step Three: Over the next seven days, focus on drinking warm water with lemon.** If you notice any changes, don't be afraid to take notes in the space provided below. These can help you have added motivation later. Ask yourself the following questions as the week progresses:

a. How do I feel?

_____

_____

_____

b. What has changed?

_____

_____

_____

c. How does my body feel?

_____

_____

_____

_____

SELF-CARE

One of the most difficult habits for my clients to start is often self-care. Women, especially, seem to find it harder to take time for themselves. We are so used to making room for everyone else but us.

Self-care is the most fun nourishing habit to start!

Self-care is different for everyone. What may look like self-care to me may not be self-care for you, which is why it's so important to tailor this habit to what really fills you—and then be flexible. What worked for you a few months ago may not work now. Don't be afraid to be creative. Just like all the nourishing habits in this book, your version of self-care will look different than someone else's. Make sure that it fills you up, whatever it is.

This week is going to be a little different in structuring your new nourishing habit. Instead of giving you three options to choose from, we're going to simplify. Set a goal to do one act of self-care every day. Test different ideas, if you want. Maybe you *think* something will be self-care, but you find out it's more draining than filling. Figure out why it didn't work.

Use the ideas listed below to get you started, then put seven different things, one on each day, in your calendar. I've given you room to fill in your own ideas at the bottom.

- Taking yourself out to dinner.
- Hiring a babysitter.
- Going to a movie.

- Going on a date with your partner.
- Having a spa day.
- Getting a manicure or pedicure.
- Paying someone else to prepare your meals.
- Sitting on the couch at the end of the day in total silence.
- Renting a car you've always wanted to drive.

- Going on vacation.
- Cutting toxic people out of your life.
- Trying a new recipe.
- Buying a new outfit.
- Making a new friend.
- Going on a first date.
- _____
- _____
- _____
- _____

Once you're done testing the new nourishing habit, there's space to make a new plan for the next week.

Working Through the Steps

1. **Step One: What initial change works for you?**
   a. Schedule the self-care into your day. Don't "hope" you make it happen.
   b. Involve anyone that's part of your daily life. They can help you be successful.
   c. Start with fifteen minutes of self-care at a time, and work up to longer.
   d. _____
   e. _____
   f. _____

2. **Step Two: Replace old habits.**

   a. What are your old habits?

   _____

   _____

   b. What will you replace them with?

   _____

   _____

   c. How will this change positively benefit you?

   _____

   _____

3. **Step Three: Over the next seven days, focus on your self-care routine.** If you notice any changes, don't be afraid to take notes in the space provided below. These can help you have added motivation later. Ask yourself the following questions as the week progresses:

   a. How do I feel?

   _____

   _____

   b. What has changed?

   _____

   _____

   _____

c. How does my body feel?

_____

_____

_____

_____

DRINK 8-10 GLASSES OF WATER A DAY

Start thinking about water like a macronutrient—it's important, and you need to get it in every single day, or everything goes off balance. As a general rule, I tell my clients to plan on drinking about eighty ounces of water a day. If you have more, that's great. Much less and you run the risk of dehydration or other problems.

Pick one of the suggestions below, and implement it as a nourishing habit for the next seven days. Be sure to come back and write down how you feel, as well as any feedback that you've gathered, in the space provided below. Once you're done testing the new nourishing habit, there's space to make a new plan for the next week.

1. **Set an ounces-per-day goal.** I recommend everyone have at least eighty ounces of water per day, but depending on your weight, height, and activity level, you may need more. If you live in a hot climate or exercise vigorously, aim for at least 100 ounces per day.
2. **Cut out soda.** Get more water in by making it the only beverage you consume. Cut out soda for seven days, and

replace it with water. The extra hydration can help you through the withdrawals.

3. **Replace alcohol with tea.** Turn to a hot cup of tea when you're tempted to slip into that nightly wine habit, or consider trying kombucha or mineral water. Not only will this help increase your water intake, but it cuts out the detrimental effects of alcohol as well.

Working Through the Steps

1. **Step One: What initial change works for you?**
   a. Get rid of all the soda or alcohol in your house.
   b. Buy a refillable water bottle.
   c. Invest in what you need, like an ice cube tray if you like your drinks cold, or some flavors of tea that you'd like to try or have loved in the past.
   d. _____
   e. _____
   f. _____

2. **Step Two: Replace old habits.**

   a. What are your old habits?

   _____

   _____

   b. What will you replace them with?

   _____

   _____

   c. How will this change positively benefit you?

_____

_____

_____

3. **Step Three: Over the next seven days, focus on your water intake.** If you notice any changes, don't be afraid to take notes in the space provided below. These can help you have added motivation later. Ask yourself the following questions as the week progresses:

   a. How do I feel?

_____

_____

_____

   b. What has changed?

_____

_____

_____

   c. How does my body feel?

_____

_____

_____

POSITIVE SELF-TALK

The way you speak to yourself can ultimately decide whether you're successful in implementing your new nourishing habits or not.

When those negative feelings encroach that say, "I can't do this! This is too much!" just take a deep breath, and say to yourself, "No, it's only food. (Or exercise or fasting or the scale, etc.) I like to eat this way because my body feels good this way."

These positive statements actually give you more energy. Tony Robbins has trained himself to only spend ninety seconds on a what-if thought. He allows himself to have the thought, but he doesn't stay with it.

When dealing with anxiety, one of the most beneficial things I have found is to write the anxious thoughts down in a journal. Journaling is so important! Write down your problem, then give yourself three options to solve it. There's something in the act of writing it down that helps us release it from our mind. We can look at it more objectively, and then find solutions.

Pick one of the suggestions below, and implement it as a nourishing habit for the next seven days. Be sure to come back and write down how you feel, as well as any feedback that you've gathered, in the space provided below. Once you're done testing the new nourishing habit, there's space to make a new plan for the next week.

1. **Listen to the narrative in your head.** Sometimes, the hardest part of fixing ANTS is knowing what you're saying to yourself. When you feel that anxiety or fear or pressure, stop and ask, "What are the thoughts in my head right now?"
2. **Replace the negative with positive.** When you hear something negative in your head, replace it with something positive. You can even say it out loud. For example, let's say you step on the scale, and your stomach drops at what you see. Instead of thinking *I will never lose weight,* you can say to yourself, "Weight loss is a process, and I can do this."
3. **Write affirmations every day.** As part of staying positive, write down affirmations (or positive statements) that you want to believe are true in a journal. For example, you could write down *I am always successful,* or *My body is constantly getting to better health.*

Working Through the Steps

1. **Step One: What works for you?**
   a. Establish a time to write your positive thoughts down and stick to it. I suggest in the morning, before you start your day.
   b. Say the positive thoughts out loud while driving instead of listening to the radio.
   c. Buy a special journal to fill with your positive thoughts.
   d. _____

e. ....

f. _____

2. **Step Two: Replace old habits.**

   a. What are your old habits?

   _____
   ....
   _____

   b. What will you replace them with?

   _____
   ....
   _____

   c. How will this change positively benefit you?

   _____
   ....
   _____

3. **Step Three: Over the next seven days, focus on positive self-talk.** If you notice any changes, don't be afraid to take notes in the space provided below. These can help you have added motivation later. Ask yourself the following questions as the week progresses:

   a. How do I feel?

   _____
   ....
   _____
   ....

b. What has changed?

_____

_____

_____

_____

c. How does my body feel?

_____

_____

_____

_____

FASTING

With all my clients, I like them to start fasting as simply as possible. This is another nourishing habit that we're going to do in a bit more targeted way. I want you to try this out very intentionally.

When you start fasting, plan to fast for twelve hours at night. If you want to eat breakfast at 7:00 in the morning, stop eating at 7:00 at night. Water and clear liquids (like unsweetened tea) are fine. Anything with sugar doesn't count. We want your body to be at complete digestive rest for twelve hours.

If you already do this, feel free to advance this to fourteen hours of digestive rest every day, but don't go past sixteen, particularly if you have thyroid issues. If you have other health issues, be sure to check with your doctor before proceeding.

For the first three days when you start intermittent fasting, you may feel hunger pains in your fasting window. These are normal as the body adjusts. After that, your body shifts to burn stored fat for fuel, which is definitely something we want because it aids in fat loss. Be careful you're not overdoing it and breaking down the body instead. Don't let this get out of control, backfire, and cause the body more stress.

Be sure that when you fast, you honor it appropriately. During your fast, consume nothing but water. Also, don't be afraid to experiment, test, and get feedback on what works best for your body.

Pick one of the suggestions below, and implement it as a nourishing habit for the next seven days. Be sure to come back and write down how you feel, as well as any feedback that you've gathered, in the space provided below. Once you're done testing the new nourishing habit, there's space to make a new plan for the next week.

1. **Stop eating twelve hours before you want breakfast.** This can be 7:00 in the evening, or even 9:00 (although I don't recommend eating three hours before bed if you can avoid it).

2. **Drink warm lemon water or tea in the morning.** Not only will this help you get in water and detox, but it can help stave off hunger pains that sometimes arise when you start fasting.

3. **Reassess.** If fasting was easier than you expected, go ahead and increase your fast to fourteen hours. If it was too difficult at twelve, try ten, then gradually move up from there.

Working Through the Steps

1. **Step One: What works for you?**
   a. Stop eating twelve hours before breakfast.
   b. Have tea or water ready in case you need help finishing the last hour or two of your fast.
   c. Replace your early breakfast with another habit, such as a walk, meditation, or preparing for your day.
   d. _____

e. _____

f. _____

2. **Step Two: Replace old habits.**

   a. What are your old habits?

   _____

   _____

   b. What will you replace them with?

   _____

   _____

   c. How will this change positively benefit you?

   _____

   _____

3. **Step Three: Over the next seven days, focus on fasting for at least twelve hours.** If you notice any changes, don't be afraid to take notes in the space provided below. These can help you have added motivation later. Ask yourself the following questions as the week progresses:

   a. How do I feel?

   _____

   _____

   _____

b. What has changed?

_____

_____

_____

c. How does my body feel?

_____

_____

_____

EXERCISE

Exercise can be a daunting word.

When you're starting out with this nourishing habit, I don't want you to go crazy. Working out too hard just makes our body break down, which only makes things worse!

If you currently don't exercise, I recommend starting small. Focus on gentle exercise or movement. Going on three ten-minute walks a day is a great start. You can eventually build up to walking 5-7 days a week. From there, look for hills or stairs to challenge yourself and strengthen your back side. This will help the body stay strong and minimize injury.

Any movement is great, but thirty – sixty minutes a day is ideal. Form the habit of getting out and doing it. This could be playing fris-bee, going for a stroll, taking your dog around the block, or dancing with your kids. Just get out there. Establish the habit. Gentle exercise can be one of our highest forms of self-care. You can graduate up to bigger things, like increasing your heart rate by doing stairs, lunges, or hills. Your endurance will build into something bigger. Eventually, the habit becomes easy.

If you're already someone who exercises, change it up to some-thing more challenging. Add weights for muscle bearing or try a new kind of workout. Do something different.

Pick one of the suggestions below, and implement it as a nourishing habit for the next seven days. Be sure to come back and write down how you feel, as well as any feedback that you've gathered, in the space provided below. Once you're done testing the new nourishing habit, there's space to make a new plan for the next week.

1. **Go for a walk in the morning.** This gentle exercise is easy for everyone to do, and you can scale it to your abilities. Start with ten minutes and add an extra five minutes every day.

2. **Buy a set of free weights.** There are plenty of free exercise routines online that you can do with a weight set of your choosing. It's a great way to build that calorie-burning muscle!

3. **Try something new.** Each day this week, implement a new exercise — swimming, Pilates, hiking, yoga, bike riding, gentle jogging. Then look back and figure out which one you liked the best.

Working Through the Steps

4. **Step One: What works for you?**
   a. Set an alarm to remind you to move. Plan for it to be a time of day when you could actually move around, like during your lunch break or after the kiddos are in bed.
   b. Get your family involved! Plan fun family games to play outside.
   c. Buy a pair of walking shoes that feel good and supportive so you're ready to go.

d. _____

e. _____

f. _____

5. **Step Two: Replace old habits.**

   a. What are your old habits?

   _____

   _____

   b. What will you replace them with?

   _____

   _____

   c. How will this change positively benefit you?

   _____

   _____

   _____

6. **Step Three: Over the next seven days, focus on your exercise.** If you notice any changes, don't be afraid to take notes in the space provided below. These can help you have added motivation later. Ask yourself the following questions as the week progresses:

   a. How do I feel?

   _____

   _____

   _____

b. What has changed?

c. How does my body feel?

BALANCE YOUR MACROS

Balancing your macros at each meal sets you up for health and food success from the very first bite. Keep your focus this week on making sure that there is fat, a fibrous vegetable, and protein on your plate every time you eat. These contain all the fiber, vitamins, and minerals you need to be healthy.

Before diving into a meal this week, ask yourself:

1. Will this fuel my body?
2. Will it give me energy?
3. Will it drain my energy?
4. Will it fight disease or cause disease?

Being intentional about what you eat and how you want to feel will help you seek out nutrients to nourish your body.

Pick one of the suggestions below, and implement it as a nourishing habit for the next seven days. Be sure to come back and write down how you feel, as well as any feedback that you've gathered, in the space provided below. Once you're done testing the new nourishing habit, there's space to make a new plan for the next week.

1. **Focus on healthy fats.** Swap vegetable oil, butter, or lard for coconut oil, avocado oil, and olive oil.
2. **Try a new vegetable.** Be adventurous when you balance your macros! Try new vegetables so you're sure that you're getting the fiber your body needs.
3. **Plan your meals ahead of time.** It seems like a daunting task to plan out a week of meals and make a grocery list, but being prepared makes balancing your macros a breeze. I provide resources at the back of the book to help your meal prepping adventure.

Working Through the Steps

1. **Step One: What initial change works for you?**
   a. Fill half your plate with veggies first. That will ensure you get more fiber.
   b. Eat with a plate at every meal. This means no leaning over the sink or eating while you drive. Sit down with it so you can visualize and see the macronutrients.
   c. If you want to see the breakdown and numbers, track what you're eating on an app.
   d. _____
   e. _____
   f. _____

2. **Step Two: Replace old habits.**

   a. What are your old habits?

   _____

   _____

   b. What will you replace them with?

   _____

   _____

   c. How will this change positively benefit you?

   _____

   _____

   _____

3. **Step Three: Over the next seven days, focus on balancing the macros in your meals.** If you notice any changes, don't be afraid to take notes in the space provided below. These can help you have added motivation later. Ask yourself the following questions as the week progresses:

   a. How do I feel?

   _____

   _____

   _____

   b. What has changed?

   _____

   _____

   _____

c. How does my body feel?

_____

....

_____

....

LIMIT YOUR STRESS

Decreasing stress is easier than it may seem. We tend to hold on to a lot of things (and beliefs) that we really don't need. This nourishing habit is all about challenging those ideas and letting go.

Where possible, create less focus on things. Use your journal to write out things that are bothering you, or vent when you're upset. Sometimes just changing your environment, or putting on music, can go a long way.

This week, let go of expectations that don't serve you. We spend so much time taking care of everyone else, we rarely do it for ourselves. When we do something good for ourselves, we feel refreshed and ready to take on more. You know how you feel when you're renewed and rejuvenated? Fight for that feeling this week. The stress can melt away.

Pick one of the suggestions below, and implement it as a nourishing habit for the next seven days. Be sure to come back and write down how you feel, as well as any feedback that you've gathered, in the space provided below. Once you're done testing the new nourishing habit, there's space to make a new plan for the next week.

1. **Get more rest.** This doesn't have to be sleep (although that helps too.) Watching a movie, laying on your

couch, or doing a puzzle can help your body have some downtime. Schedule it into your day if you have to.

2. **Breathe deep.** Sit, relax, and focus on taking deep breaths. Start at five minutes and work up from there. Or just breathe for as long as you need it. Your breath is one of your biggest allies with stress management. Being aware of our breath can help us lower our stressful defenses. It helps our body physically relax as well.

3. **Reduce caffeine.** This can make us feel more stressed out and drained, so cutting out caffeine is a first line defense in reducing stress.

Working Through the Steps

1. **Step One: What initial change works for you?**
   a. Schedule a massage, pedicure, facial, or something that feels equally as de-stressing to you.
   b. Offload two chores you do at home to someone else, then pay attention to how you feel after. Are you more stressed? Less stressed? Why?
   c. Do a session of yoga or meditation every morning to start your day. Double bonus if you do it before you go to bed, too!
   d. ....
   e. _____
   f. ....

2. **Step Two: Replace old habits.**

   a. What are your old habits?

   _____

   _____

   b. What will you replace them with?

   _____

   _____

   c. How will this change positively benefit you?

   _____

   _____

   _____

3. **Step Three: Over the next seven days, focus on your de-stressing routine.** If you notice any changes, don't be afraid to take notes in the space provided below. These can help you have added motivation later. Ask yourself the following questions as the week progresses:

   a. How do I feel?

   _____

   _____

   _____

   b. What has changed?

   _____

   _____

   _____

   _____

c. How does my body feel?

_____

....

_____

....

NOURISHING HABIT #11:

KEEP YOUR INSULIN DOWN

When we think about managing your insulin through nourishing your body, the goal is to avoid grazing all day long. Eating all the time keeps your insulin and blood sugar levels high. It doesn't allow your gut to have any rest or downtime.

Pick one of the suggestions below, and implement it as a nourishing habit for the next seven days. Be sure to come back and write down how you feel, as well as any feedback that you've gathered, in the space provided below. Once you're done testing the new nourishing habit, there's space to make a new plan for the next week.

1. **Stop snacking.** Despite recent trends that tell us to snack all day long, the truth is that our body doesn't need a constant flow of food. In fact, we're more likely to change our body mass index if we don't eat in between meals.[64] This week, I want you to make sure you're having three meals and nothing in between. If you need a snack, limit them.

2. **Write down what you eat.** People that journal tend to meet greater success. Tracking what you're eating (and when) brings awareness. There are a lot of ways you can

track or journal your food. I recommend any of these apps: MyFitnessPal, Lose It, or Carb Manager. You could even just use the notes section in your phone or a regular piece of paper.

3. **Cut out processed sugar**. You don't need it, and it's the fastest way to start seeing a change. Choose foods that have more fiber and a lower carbohydrate count. High carbohydrate foods, particularly filled with processed sugar, are the foods that stimulate secretion of insulin the most. Cut the carbs, lower your insulin, and you'll start to eat less automatically (and without as much hunger!)

Working Through the Steps

1. **Step One: What initial change works for you?**
   a. Get rid of all your snacky, sugary foods, particularly the ones you reach for in the afternoon, if your energy dips.
   b. Don't focus on one single part of your plate—like calories or carbohydrates. Do you need more fiber? What kind of fats are you mostly consuming? This will keep you aware of the bigger picture.
   c. Write down your energy levels on a scale of 1-10 throughout the day. Pay attention to how your energy changes based on the foods you eat.
   d. _____
   e. _____
   f. _____

2. **Step Two: Replace old habits.**

   a. What are your old habits?

   _____

   _____

   _____

   b. What will you replace them with?

   _____

   _____

   _____

   c. How will this change positively benefit you?

   _____

   _____

   _____

3. **Step Three: Over the next seven days, focus on keeping your insulin down.** If you notice any changes, don't be afraid to take notes in the space provided below. These can help you have added motivation later. Ask yourself the following questions as the week progresses:

   a. How do I feel?

   _____

   _____

   _____

   b. What has changed?

   _____

   _____

   _____

c. How does my body feel?

_____

_____

_____

_____

_____

CELEBRATE YOUR WINS

One of the best parts of nourishing yourself is throwing a little party for all the wins you have! Women, in particular, tend to underestimate the good things they do. My clients focus on the ways they're failing, or comparing themselves to others. Getting into the soul-nourishing habit of celebrating when you've accomplished something, no matter how big or small, can truly feed your body and soul.

Pick one of the suggestions below, and implement it as a nourishing habit for the next seven days. Be sure to come back and write down how you feel, as well as any feedback that you've gathered, in the space provided below. Once you're done testing the new nourishing habit, there's space to make a new plan for the next week.

1. **Write down five wins every day.** You can do this on a paper on your fridge so you see it every day, or in a special notebook. Don't be afraid to literally celebrate—go have a dance party!

2. **Share your wins for the day with another person.** If it helps you to be accountable and get feedback, make celebrating your wins a nightly habit with your partner, friend, or children. Maybe they'll do the same!

3. **Stop comparing yourself.** Get off of social media for a week. Is it easier for you to celebrate yourself?

Working Through the Steps

1. **Step One: What initial change works for you?**
    a. Buy a notebook or grab a piece of paper you can see every day. Seeing all your previous wins will only help you feel better!
    b. Remove your social media apps from your phones. Replace that time with a review of your wins for that day.
    c. Have a party! Dance in the kitchen, make your favorite meal, or tell your team at work, and let them join you. Get creative!
    d. _____
    e. _____
    f. _____

2. **Step Two: Replace old habits.**

    a. What are your old habits?

    _____

    _____

    b. What will you replace them with?

    _____

    _____

c. How will this change positively benefit you?

_____

_____

_____

3. **Step Three: Over the next seven days, focus on celebrating your wins.** If you notice any changes, don't be afraid to take notes in the space provided below. These can help you have added motivation later. Ask yourself the following questions as the week progresses:

a. How do I feel?

_____

_____

_____

b. What has changed?

_____

_____

_____

c. How does my body feel?

_____

_____

_____

LOSE WEIGHT

Weight loss is different for every person, which is why one single habit may not make all the difference in your weight loss efforts. In combination, however, the power of many nourishing habits is unparalleled!

In approaching this habit, I want you to focus on the nourishing habits, and have faith that weight loss will come. If we come from a place where we're really nurturing our body, and we're good to it, then the weight is going to release. And it's going to release more easily!

This week will address habits that specifically help you lose more weight. Because this is an issue that I work on with almost all of my clients, this week will also be a little different. I provide several nourishing habits below for you to pick from.

Nourishing Habit Ideas for Losing Weight

- Eat a high-protein breakfast. It has been shown to reduce cravings and calorie intake throughout the day.
- Avoid sugary drinks and fruit juice. These are the most fattening things you can put into your body because of the insulin response it triggers.

- Drink water a half hour before meals. It's well understood that drinking water before meals reduces the amount of food you eat.[65]
- Eat vegetables and fruits because they are high in fiber and micronutrients.
- Avoid alcohol.
- Eat mostly whole, unprocessed foods, which are healthier, more filling, and much less likely to cause overeating.
- Eat your food slowly. Fast eaters gain more weight over time.[66] Eating slowly makes you feel more full and boosts weight-reducing hormones.
- Use smaller plates. It works! One study shows[67] that people eat more when they use larger plates.

Working Through the Steps

1. **Step One: What initial change works for you?**
   a. Grab a small plate first—this will help you naturally plate less and pay more attention to what you're getting.
   b. Serve up your veggies first.
   c. Eat only from your plate, not other people's plates.
   d. ....
   e. _____
   f. ....

2. **Step Two: Replace old habits.**

a. What are your old habits?

_____

_____

_____

b. What will you replace them with?

_____

_____

_____

c. How will this change positively benefit you?

_____

_____

_____

3. **Step Three: Over the next seven days, focus on losing weight.** If you notice any changes, don't be afraid to take notes in the space provided below. These can help you have added motivation later. Ask yourself the following questions as the week progresses:

a. How do I feel?

_____

_____

_____

b. What has changed?

_____

_____

_____

c. How does my body feel?

_____

....

_____

....

GIVE YOURSELF GRACE

This is the final habit on purpose. After you've worked through all of these, I want you to have learned, created a better relationship with yourself, and most of all, figured out how to give yourself grace.

This process was never meant to help you achieve perfection. It's all about creating nourishing habits that enable you to create safety in your everyday life. That means sometimes you may crash a little. Willpower will fade. Motivation comes and goes. But these habits can remain . . . if you learn to give yourself grace.

Pick one of the suggestions below, and implement it as a nourishing habit for the next seven days. Be sure to come back and write down how you feel, as well as any feedback that you've gathered, in the space provided below. Once you're done testing the new nourishing habit, there's space to make a new plan for the next week.

1. **Let go of perfection.** Every day, think back on what didn't go as well as you expected, then let go of the things that didn't go perfectly.
2. **Figure out your feedback.** At night, think through things that went well first, then look at what didn't. What does that feedback tell you? What can you do differently tomorrow?
3. **Release expectations.** Some of my clients barrel into

their day with a to-do list a million miles long, then get frustrated when it's incomplete (or bigger!) by bedtime. Release your expectations of the day, and let it flow.

Working Through the Steps

1. **Step One: What initial change works for you?**
   a. Use meditation to release expectations for the day.
   b. Speak your release out loud. Say, "I give myself grace to be human and imperfect," every day.
   c. Write down what you learned from your day, both good and bad. What can you do differently?
   d. _____
   e. _____
   f. _____

2. **Step Two: Replace old habits.**

   a. What are your old habits?

   _____

   _____

   _____

   b. What will you replace them with?

   _____

   _____

   _____

   c. How will this change positively benefit you?

   _____

   _____

   _____

3. **Step Three: Over the next seven days, focus on giving yourself grace.** If you notice any changes, don't be afraid to take notes in the space provided below. These can help you have added motivation later. Ask yourself the following questions as the week progresses:

a. How do I feel?

b. What has changed?

c. How does my body feel?

Ideas for a successful new habit:

1. _____

2. _____

3. _____

Start date:

Working Through the New Habit Steps

1. **Step One: What initial change works for you?**

   a. _____

   b. _____

   c. _____

2. **Step Two: Replace old habits.**

   a. What are your old habits?

   _____

   _____

   _____

b. What will you replace them with?

c. How will this change positively benefit you?

3. **Step Three: Over the next seven days, focus on your new routine.** If you notice any changes, don't be afraid to take notes in the space provided below. These can help you have added motivation later. Ask yourself the following questions as the week progresses:

a. How do I feel?

b. What has changed?

c. How does my body feel?

Ideas for a successful new habit:

1. _____

2. _____

3. _____

Start date:

Working Through the New Habit Steps

1. **Step One: What initial change works for you?**

   a. _____

   b. _____

   c. _____

2. **Step Two: Replace old habits.**

   a. What are your old habits?

   _____

   _____

   _____

b. What will you replace them with?

_____

_____

_____

c. How will this change positively benefit you?

_____

_____

_____

3. **Step Three: Over the next seven days, focus on your new routine.** If you notice any changes, don't be afraid to take notes in the space provided below. These can help you have added motivation later. Ask yourself the following questions as the week progresses:

a. How do I feel?

_____

_____

_____

b. What has changed?

_____

_____

_____

c. How does my body feel?

_____

_____

_____

Ideas for a successful new habit:

1. _____

2. _____

3. _____

Start date:

Working Through the New Habit Steps

1. **Step One: What initial change works for you?**

   a. _____

   b. _____

   c. _____

2. **Step Two: Replace old habits.**

   a. What are your old habits?

   _____

   _____

   _____

b. What will you replace them with?

_____

_____

_____

c. How will this change positively benefit you?

_____

_____

_____

3. **Step Three: Over the next seven days, focus on your new routine.** If you notice any changes, don't be afraid to take notes in the space provided below. These can help you have added motivation later. Ask yourself the following questions as the week progresses:

a. How do I feel?

_____

_____

_____

b. What has changed?

_____

_____

_____

c. How does my body feel?

_____

_____

_____

PUTTING IT ALL TOGETHER

Choosing to get healthy is one of the best decisions you can make.

Whether you want to lose weight or get healthier, there is no better time than now! When you become healthier, everyone around you benefits. Your body is the only place you have to live, so take care of it. You can do that best through the nourishing habits.

When you implement your nourishing habits, I want them to help you to look at nourishing your body and soul differently. Instead of looking at food as an emotional crutch or safety net, I want you to see food as fuel and nourishment. Instead of looking to alcohol as pleasure or comfort, find a way to give your body what it needs. If you only had one car for the rest of your life, you'd take care of it and give it all the good things it needs. Your body is no different! If you want it to last a long time, take care of it. At 4:00 p.m., your body doesn't need coffee, a Danish, or a glass of wine!

Think of your nourishing habits this way: if you could have a conversation with your body, what would it ask you for?

What is your body trying to tell you?

Is it your gut that needs a little bit more love?

Are you dealing with daily headaches? Brittle nails and dry skin?

If we start paying attention, we can heal our bodies one symptom at a time. How amazing would you feel if you didn't have the burden of feeling unhealthy, or exhausted, or hungover? My goal is to help you treat the problem, not the symptom. Oftentimes, we are our biggest problem! As you work through the nourishing habits in this book over and over, ask yourself, *what has my body been telling me?*

What's eating *you*?

What feels easy enough for you to do right now?

What do you want the most?

Start today by loving yourself unconditionally. Love all the wrinkles, gray hair, cellulite, and perceived imperfections. Remember that no one is perfect. You can keep going even though it may not feel like it, because the best plan to be on is the consistent one.

Consistency doesn't mean never messing up, it means never *giving* up.

Focus on how you feel, not just the scale. Let's focus on getting strong. Let's focus on getting healthy so it gives you the power to get what you want. You can't pour from an empty cup, which is why nourishing our soul is so important. You need to fill *you* up. You need to love yourself period. You need to be your own cheerleader. You'll come from a good place, which helps you handle stress better, have more fun, and be more confident.

The need for nourishing habits that apply across the board for anyone to try is why I'm bringing you this book now, at a time when information is overabundant and the market saturated with gurus. My plan is simple, involves your body telling you what is best for you, and then you establishing healthy habits to help you succeed.

Keep going, and don't give up. Eventually, you will get there. When you put in the work, things can change. You can change your own life, create the world that you want, and be more available to fulfill your dreams.

I know you can do this.

If you need any extra support, I invite you to reach out to me at info.nourishyourbody@gmail.com. Working with women to bring greater nourishment and health is my life passion.

PART FIVE

ADDITIONAL
Resources

TROUBLESHOOTING
WEIGHT LOSS

What if this doesn't work? I'm sure you're asking yourself that—I ask myself that sometimes too. If you've been implementing my nourishing habits (and abiding by the 80/20 rule) and you just aren't seeing any changes, don't worry. There are still plenty of things we can troubleshoot or change.

If you're struggling to lose weight, go through and ask yourself the questions below. Study your response to determine if you can improve in one area. For example, if you're focusing only on the scale to check your weight loss success, what other progress indicators can you find?

Don't be afraid to revisit this list as you continue in your journey. Ask yourself the following questions:

4. Am I only focusing on the scale?
5. Am I eating too many calories?
6. Am I eating too few calories?
7. Am I exercising enough?
8. Am I exercising too much?
9. Have I tried safely lifting weights to help tone my body?
10. Have I been slipping back into eating low fat or diet foods?

11. Am I overestimating how much I work out and eating too much to compensate?
12. Am I eating enough protein?
13. Has my sleep changed recently?
14. What is my energy level?
15. What foods have I been eating lately?
16. Have I been tracking my food?
17. Have I had enough water?
18. Have I had too much caffeine?
19. Have I had too much sodium?
20. Have I had too much sugar?
21. Have I had too much alcohol?
22. Have I been battling cravings?
23. Is there too much stress in my life right now?

Below, I've listed a few tweaks you can make (or initiate into your day as nourishing habits) that may help you kick start your weight loss again. Sometimes the scale doesn't move because it's like your body wants to trust you, and that may take time. Consistency can create that environment! Oftentimes when I work with clients, we see big results with small changes over time.

Remember, it's important to start with a clean slate. This means taking the time to clean out your refrigerator and pantry. Get rid of trigger foods, processed foods, and unhealthy foods. Make room for fresh, healthy foods.

- Add protein to your diet at each meal.
- Track what you're eating.
- Check your portion sizes.
- Eat whole, single-ingredient foods.

- Avoid processed foods.
- Stock up on healthy foods and snacks.
- Limit your intake of added sugar.
- Drink water.
- Drink unsweetened coffee.
- Avoid liquid calories.
- Limit sugary carbohydrates.
- Increase your vegetable intake.
- Count calories twice a week as a "check in".
- Eat from smaller plates.
- Count carbs twice a week as a "check in".
- Eat eggs or protein for breakfast.
- Eat slowly.
- Pay closer attention to your portion size.
- Take a medical-grade quality probiotic.
- Check in with your sleep.
- Track your daily intake of fiber.
- Brush your teeth after eating to avoid snacking.
- Do low-impact cardio.
- Increase your resistance exercise.
- Stop eating processed sugar for seven days to kill off candida—then see how you feel. Has anything changed?
- Stop feeding your cravings. When you experience one, find something else to do or have, like a cup of tea or vacuum your house.
- Go for a walk, drink a big glass of water, or if you feel like you have to eat something because the craving is strong, eat something like hard boiled eggs or almonds.

The Benefits of Fruits and Veggies for Weight Loss

When trying to lose weight, make sure you're using fruits and vegetables to your advantage. Women need at least 25 grams a day of fiber. Fiber helps us get rid of toxins and feel full. To help achieve this goal, your veggies need to fill half the plate. Here are a few ways to take advantage of all the nourishing benefits:

1. Cut back on your cereal and, add berries or nuts to your bowl.
2. Add veggies to your morning egg dish.
3. Throw extra veggies into your soup instead of noodles.
4. Replace chips with raw, fresh veggies.
5. Instead of grains, eat fibrous veggies, like roasted Brussels sprouts or broccoli.
6. Avoid the vending machine, and grab a banana, an apple, or a few nuts.
7. Avoid dried fruit because of the high sugar content.
8. Avoid fruit juice. You lose the benefit of the fiber in the juice.[68]
9. Sneak vegetables in everything.
10. Drink green juice on an empty stomach.

Also keep in mind the benefits of antioxidants that fruits and vegetables provide. Antioxidants, which are substances that may delay cell death and disease, include supplements such as beta-carotene, luteine, lycopene, vitamins A, D, E, and K, and many more. Decades of research says that antioxidants may prevent or delay some types of cell damage,[69] and can have some effect on certain types of cancer.[70]

If you've been implementing these changes but see no results, or don't feel any better (like increased energy, tolerance, decreased appetite, or better sleep), all hope is not lost. There are a few more things you can look into with the help of your naturopathic doctor that may help you work through these problems.

Look over this checklist before your appointment. Make sure to bring your notes from your book along, as well as a list of questions or symptoms you have. Most of the time, symptoms are signs that something isn't working, which gives us a clue that we need to get something checked.

Suspected Medical Issue:

- **Thyroid Issues**
  - **Hypothyroid.** This is also known as *underactive thyroid* and is a condition of the thyroid gland, which is a butterfly shaped organ in your neck. Hypothyroidism can lead to weight gain and a slow metabolism.
  - **Hyperthyroid.** This is also known as an *overactive thyroid*. Most people tend to lose weight with this form of thyroid disorder, but some people may gain weight because it increases appetite so much.
- **Polycystic ovarian or ovary syndrome (PCOS).** This is a hormone disorder in women when an excess of male hormones (androgen) can cause irregular periods, facial

hair, and acne. It often causes difficulty with weight loss, or appears after excessive weight gain.

- **PMS** (premenstrual syndrome)
- **Cardiovascular diseases**
- **Diabetes.** Both types of diabetes require strict attention to blood sugar and insulin levels to keep weight gain and health at optimal levels.
  - **Type 1.** This type requires lifelong insulin level care and cannot be treated with medication.
  - **Type 2.** Long-term maintenance of blood sugar and weight loss makes this type more treatable.

TRACKING YOUR FOOD

Writing down what you eat is another way to hold yourself account-able to healthy habits and gain some feedback on what you're doing. All of my most successful clients track what they're eating. That can be in a journal, on an app, or a piece of paper tacked to your fridge. The accountability helps us make better decisions, and the data in-forms our future decisions as well. My favorite phone apps are Carb Manager, MyFitnessPal, and Lose It.

What I love about tracking your food is the visibility you gain. You can see how much you're eating and can track your nutrient breakdown also. This helps you have a better picture of what's really going on. Here's a few things you can track (or ask yourself) if you're having trouble with weight loss and can't figure out why.

1. How many grams of sugar do you consume?
2. Is it higher on the weekend? Why?
3. What's your cholesterol intake?
4. Fiber?
5. What's your calorie intake?
6. Protein?
7. Healthy fats?
8. Minerals?

While I don't advocate for intense calorie restriction, there can come a time when we need to cut back the amount we're consuming. You can be eating great macros, but still be getting too much food. Even healthy food can make us gain weight! One of my clients who struggled to lose weight approached me in some frustration. When we went over her food, we discovered that she ate two avocados a day on top of everything else. Avocados are great—but they can add up!

Paying attention to how much you're eating can create a lot of visibility. "Julie," my client Debbie said during one of our calls. "I just *can't* lose weight. I'm eating great. I'm doing what you tell me. The scale just won't budge."

This young woman was right—she did everything I told her to. Even I felt a little perplexed. Her scale should have been moving. Deciding that we needed a bit more visibility into her actual eating process, I said, "This week, I want you to focus on tracking your food. You've done a great job cutting out processed foods, but let's see if something else is going on."

The next week, Debbie hopped back on a call. She'd sent me pictures of her food log, and we went through them together. Writing down what she was eating revealed a *very* interesting picture! While eating healthy, Debbie had turned to some form of nuts for almost all her snacks. She ate peanut butter by the spoonful. While watching television, she would sit down with a tin of nuts and snack. When she didn't have that, handfuls of almonds, some healthy trail mix, bars, and more populated her lists.

"I see the problem!" I said. "You are eating better foods, but it's almost all from one food group and way too many calories. We need to cut back on the nuts!"

This is a common scenario with some of my clients, who tend to be sensitive to nuts and their higher calories. Without tracking, however, I wouldn't have been able to analyze what was going on for Debbie. This story also reiterates the fact that there is no failure, only feedback. Debbie took the feedback, made some changes, and the scale started to move!

Nutrients like fiber and cholesterol are rarely as emphasized as calories or carbs or fat, but those are important nutrients as well. Depending on your current health and family history, they can be very important to track. When used correctly, tracking is a good feedback tool. Just like Debbie, writing down what you're eating may surprise you!

MEAL PREPPING

Introducing the idea of meal prepping sometimes meets resistance with my clients, but it is one of the biggest determinants of success in the women I work with.

It's so worth it!

That's why I'm creating a guide. Not only is it a good habit to get into, but it will help you be successful with many nourishing habits, like eating balanced macros or limiting stress. Meal prepping can really decreases your stress.

Let's dive more into this.

Meal Prepping to Success

Having a strategy around meal preparation immediately sets you up for success. Not only does it take the guesswork out, but the time too. You don't have to waste energy wondering what you're going to fix for dinner. If you leave for the grocery store without a list, you could forget something or buy a lot of junk. Plus, it can be as simple as taking the time to think meals over the day before.

"Julie," my client, Abby, said to me one day, "I know you really want me to meal prep, but that just seems *so big*."

We were ending an hour-long call, for part of which she and I had discussed the difficulty of her living situation. Because she lived more than forty-five minutes from a grocery store or a fast-food restaurant, the burden of meals on her was heavier than most of my clients. She literally had to fix everything—there was no quick trip to the store to grab a rotisserie chicken! Despite living so far away, she didn't really organize her food system and often lamented about how frustrating it was to budget, fix, and decide her meals for a small family of four.

"I know," I told her. "Meal prepping does seem big. But I promise it's worth it. What do you hate more than anything?"

At this, she groaned. "Deciding what to make for dinner. It hangs on me some days, and the last thing I want to do is open the fridge and figure it out."

"And we just spoke about setting yourself up for success, right?"

"Right."

"Meal prepping will do it. It's easier than you think, I promise."

Not only did Abby give it a try—she ended up loving it. She scheduled a trip to a wholesale store, loaded up on her favorite veggies and meats, then came home and spent two hours on meal prep. She put food away, sliced raw chicken, bagged it, labeled it for the fridge. What she didn't cut into portions and freeze, she had cooking in the background. After organizing her system, she sent me a picture over text. Inside her fridge waited fifteen ready-to-go meals.

When we hopped on a call and discussed her experience, the feedback was *very* different.

"I can't believe it," she said. "I don't have to think about what I'm going to eat for the rest of the week. Even though I had to have it going for two hours, it's definitely saved me time now. It's so easy, Julie. So easy."

It really is! In theory, meal prepping may seem like it's difficult or a large time commitment, but it's all in how you approach it. You don't have to go all-in like Abby. You can simply get into the habit of slicing, cutting, or chopping veggies once you get home from the grocery store so they're ready to go.

Imagine how good it feels to open your refrigerator and have all your meals prepared! Not to mention the power of removing decisions. Instead of having to remember to pull meat out of the freezer or stop by the grocery store on your way home, it's already done. Otherwise you may wait too long to get something to eat and end up battling the ghrelin monster. Or let's say you didn't meal prep. At the end of a long day, you open your fridge to realize that you only have cheese and tortillas.

Picture that day.

You're on a roll at work and at home. Everything is going great, you're knocking out tons on your list and want to maintain your steady momentum. It's lunchtime, so you reach for what you have . . . and it isn't much. Or it requires elaborate time preparation you can't commit to right then.

What will you do? Probably reach for food that isn't that great for you, or skip your meal and end up battling the ghrelin monster at dinner. (And we all know what that looks like!) Meal prepping can truly set you up for success and keep your motivation high because you're ready. If you're still feeling resistance to meal prepping, let's dive a little deeper and question what feels normal to you.

What's getting in your way?

Why don't you have time?

Why can't you take two hours on a weekend to save you hours (not to mention stress) during the week?

Is it really *that* hard?

I love to post on my Instagram account what it cost to make my meals, which are all organic, so follow me there if you want some more tips. (My handle is @nourish_nutrition) My goal is to make everything under $20 for a family of four. That is way less than picking up dinner out, which would be closer to $40! When you plan ahead, you actually save money because there is less waste. Planning will also help you figure out what to do with those leftover veggies that you never got around to using. They are perfect to put in an egg casserole or soup . . . and super easy!

Meal prepping is one of the most beneficial ways to save yourself some time and mental energy. In the long run, planning is easier. From meal plans, prepping the food, scheduling time to go to the grocery store every week, to creating your shopping list before you go. It's easier to be successful that way. If it's on our calendar, we'll probably do it.

How to Meal Prep

1. Choose a day of the week that makes the most sense for you to do meal planning or prep. Is it Monday after the weekend? Saturday evening? Sunday afternoon before the week starts? Find that day, and commit to it. When it becomes a habit, you'll naturally fall into it every week.
2. Make a list of five to six of your favorite dinners.
3. Now write down all the groceries you need for those dinners.
4. Make a list of healthy snacks (but not too many!) that you want to keep around the house for those days when you need *a little something*.

5. Schedule time on your calendar to go to the store, come home, and put at least three meals together.
6. Go to the store, and buy those groceries.
7. Prep the meals at home according to your schedule for that week. Prepping can be as simple as cutting and bagging the veggies, or it may mean preparing a casserole that you put into the freezer to use later.
8. Step back and enjoy the delicious feeling of not having to worry about what you're going to eat through the week!

Tips for Meal Prepping

1. Plan before you get to the grocery store so you know exactly what to buy, and how much. Not only does this prevent you from buying things that aren't good for you, but it will help you have a tighter budget as well.
2. Buy washable containers that will be easy to reuse and stack in your refrigerator. I like glass if possible. I try not to use or recommend using plastic. The polycarbons can seep into our foods and increase our estrogen.
3. Some weeks are busier than others. For those times when you can't pull it all together, consider a meal delivery service. Ones that have full meals already cooked are ideal (otherwise you need to plan meal prep into your time because some meal delivery services don't make the meal, just provide the ingredients).
4. Make different meals every week so you can vary it up and not get tired of what's already prepared.

5. Schedule a recurring time slot every week, or two weeks if that best fits your life, to go back to the grocery store. That way you always know when you're going, how much food to buy, and you'll always have good food on hand.

6. Have a list of meals that you enjoy eating (or your family enjoys) with the needed ingredients before you go to the store. Keep them on your fridge if seeing them will help.

7. Cutting up food counts as well—you don't have to actually assemble the meals. Consider making your own trail mix and storing it in small, ready-to-go containers you can take with you.

8. When you're making dinner, make big batches of food, and freeze the leftovers, or have them for lunch the next day.

9. Don't forget your slow cooker! When you meal prep, you can freeze uncooked food, then pull it out in the morning, throw it in the slow cooker, turn it on, and be ready to go when you return.

10. If your budget allows, hire someone to do it for you!

FOOD LIST

When it comes to eating the right foods, we need all the help we can get, which is why I'm including this food list. Use it as a resource when you need dinner ideas (like before you go shopping, or if you don't know what to fix for dinner). Better yet, use this as your shopping list when you go to the store.

Protein Sources

- Meat—Grass fed beef, organic chicken, turkey, lamb, nitrate-free sausage
- Fish and seafood—wild salmon, shrimp, white fish
- Eggs—Omega-3 pastured raised eggs are best
- Vegan sources—tempeh, lentils, chickpeas, almonds, spirulina, quinoa, and beans
- Protein powder

Vegetables:

- Broccoli
- Cauliflower
- Spinach
- Kale
- Brussels Sprouts
- Cabbage
- Swiss Chard
- Lettuce

- Cucumber
- Celery
- Bell peppers
- Sweet potatoes
- Asparagus
- Carrots
- Zucchini
- Spaghetti squash
- Artichokes
- Eggplant
- Peas
- Beets
- Bok choy
- Snow/snap peas

Fruit:

- Blueberries
- Blackberries
- Strawberries
- Raspberries
- Apples
- Bananas
- Oranges
- Grapefruit
- Pineapple
- Papaya
- Mangos
- Apricots
- Plums
- Pears
- Grapes
- Peaches
- Lemons
- Cherries
- Kiwis

Fat Sources:

- Olive oil
- Coconut oil
- Avocado oil
- Grass-fed butter
- Ghee
- Olives
- Wild salmon
- Nuts
- Seeds
- Flax seeds
- Chia seeds
- Avocados
- Full fat dairy

Foods to Avoid or Limit

- Margarine
- Alcohol
- Canned tomatoes
- Processed meats
- Vegetable oils
- Microwave popcorn
- Sugary beverages
- Processed Foods
- Unfermented soy products
- High-fructose corn syrup
- Artificial sweetener

Focusing on healthy, protein-rich foods is always ideal. If possible, avoid foods like pastries, candy, corn sweeteners, white sugar, and brown sugar. Also be sure to avoid or limit the following foods:

Coffee

Coffee can contain over 200 pesticides in a single cup. The body puts on fat to protect its organs from toxic substances, so coffee can actually be very fattening!

If you *must* have coffee—although I encourage people to stay away from it—choose organic, roasted, whole bean coffee. Drink it black made with a non-bleached filter in the mornings before your workouts. If you are someone who skips breakfast and only drinks coffee until lunch, eat breakfast before you have coffee.

Roasted coffee prevents your stomach from producing excess acid, so darker roast coffee may be easier on your stomach than lighter roast coffee. If you have an issue with decreased adrenal function, use coffee with care, as it can be hard on your adrenal glands. Coffee also has a diuretic effect, so if you have problems with electrolyte imbalance, I suggest you avoid it.

Salt

Your body needs salt to regulate your blood pressure, help your brain communicate with your muscles, and support the function of your adrenal glands. However, your body doesn't need large amounts of processed table salt to perform optimally.

Instead, I recommend using a mixture of table salt and pink Himalayan salt. This salt is higher in potassium than any of the other natural, unprocessed salts, helping you to maintain a balanced potassium-salt ratio. The salt is very flavorful and tastes delicious on your food. You'll find that you'll need less than you do of table salt, but you'll get more flavor and more mineral content.

We still need iodine for our thyroid, which is why I don't recommend entirely cutting out table salt (which is iodized—meaning it contains iodine and helps prevent massive, widespread thyroid issues). Decreasing your use of table salt can benefit your body.

Alcohol

Simply put, alcohol can sabotage all your healthy efforts.

As soon as you have a drink, your body eats up all the glycogen (stored glucose) in your liver, makes you hungry, and reduces your inhibitions, so you're more likely to grab that chicken wing or stuffed potato skin at happy hour. Alcohol also affects the amount of B12 vitamin available for our body to use.[71]

Plus, alcoholic drinks contain many more calories than most people think. For example, a 20-ounce serving of beer can pack 250 calories, a six-ounce glass of wine contains 120 calories, and a 1.5-ounce shot of liquor contains about 100 calories. And that's without any sugary mixers.

- Beer — 250 calories
- Red or white wine — 120 calories
- Daiquiri — 259 calories
- Vodka and club soda — 64 calories
- Champagne — 84 calories
- Rum and Coke — 91 calories
- Cosmopolitan — 230 calories
- Bloody Mary — 140 calories
- Sangria — 167 calories
- Martini — 69 calories
- Margarita — 270 calories

When you drink alcohol, it gets immediate attention (because it is viewed by the body as a toxin) and needs no digestion. When the body is focused on processing alcohol, it causes your blood sugar to drop. When alcohol is consumed, it is transported to the liver where it contributes to fatty liver. The liver turns it into triglycerides, which are released into blood circulation where it can be stored as body fat.[72]

Alcohol's diuretic effect causes water loss and dehydration. Along with that, you lose important minerals, such as magnesium, potassium, calcium and zinc. These minerals are vital to the maintenance of fluid balance, chemical reactions, and muscle contraction and relaxation.

Alcohol affects your body in other negative ways. Drinking may help induce sleep, but the sleep you get isn't very deep. As a result, you get less rest, which can trigger you to eat more calories the next day. Alcohol can also increase the amount of acid that your stomach produces, causing your stomach lining to become inflamed. Over time, excessive alcohol use can lead to serious health problems, including stomach ulcers, liver disease, and heart trouble.

Alcohol can easily be the enemy when it comes to weight loss. It adds extra calories to your diet, encourages you to eat more food, and alters the normal digestive process. Not only are the extra calories a hindrance, but the changes in food breakdown turns those extra calories into unwanted body fat.

Even a few drinks a week is linked with an increased risk of breast cancer in women. This risk may be especially high in women who do not get enough folate (a B vitamin) in their diet or through supplements. Alcohol can affect estrogen levels in the body, which may explain some of the increased risk. Drinking less alcohol may be an important way for many women to lower their risk of breast cancer.

Gluten

A gluten-free diet isn't just for those with celiac disease or a wheat allergy. Although eating wheat products, especially whole wheat, does offer some health benefits, the gluten can actually be harmful. Here are some reasons you may want to consider going gluten-free.

- **Humans don't fully digest wheat.** The undigested portions of wheat begin to ferment, producing gas. Icky, belchable, fart-forming gas.
- **Wheat is a pro-inflammatory agent.** A pro-inflammatory agent is rapidly converted to sugar, causing a rise in the body's insulin levels and a burst of inflammation at the cellular level, among other problems.

- **Wheat can cause leaky gut syndrome.** Leaky gut syndrome is a condition when toxins, microbes, undigested food particles, and antibodies are leaking from your gut into your bloodstream.
- **Refined wheat has little nutritional value.** Did you know that manufacturers actually have to enrich refined wheat because they've taken out all the nutrients? And even then, the wheat's not that valuable, nutritionally speaking.
- **Wheat is one of the top-eight allergens.** Millions of people are allergic to wheat. So many, in fact, that it has made it on to the top-eight allergen list.

In fact, many people have gluten sensitivity or celiac disease and don't know it. No one knows for sure how many people this applies to, but we know that celiac disease has skyrocketed in the last fifty years. We went from 1 in 650 people having it to 1 in 120 people.[73]

ADDITIONAL NOURISHING HABITS

As you work through your new nourishing habits, I don't want you to feel stuck on the fourteen examples I provided earlier. Here are a few other nourishing habits that I've given to my clients in the past. These are here to get you thinking about what you need most and give you permission to think big. If it's adding to your health and creating safety, make it a nourishing habit!

1. Weigh-in daily or weekly.
2. Eat a good breakfast with whole foods, fiber, protein, and healthy fats.
3. Walk at least 10,000 steps a day.
4. Keep your refrigerator full. Make sure you grocery shop before it's empty.
5. Bring your own food to parties or events that you attend.
6. Plan ahead for anything, whether it's meals, trips, or parties.
7. Don't eat after 6:00 p.m. or 7:00 p.m.
8. Don't eat three hours before bedtime.

9. Read food labels. Sugar, gluten, nitrates, and other additives can hide under sneaky names or labels.
10. Let people know what you are doing. Most people want to help us be successful.
11. Eat off a smaller plate.
12. Use positive affirmations to override the negative thoughts.
13. Use a food tracking app on your phone to keep you accountable and aware.
14. Drink water all day. Don't try to catch up all at once!
15. Get rid of the trigger foods in your house. If they aren't around, you can't eat them.
16. Stock your home with healthy foods.
17. Stay home more instead of eating out because it's easy.
18. Eat smaller portions.
19. Use a journal to write down your emotions, especially when you want to eat when you're not hungry.
20. Find an accountability partner.

VITAMINS
AND
SUPPLEMENTS

Ideally, we receive our nutrients directly from the food and minerals we eat, but most of the time we're not. Most of us aren't rotating our food like we should, so we eat the same things over and over. If we have a lot of gut bacteria, we also may not absorb our nutrients like we should, which creates the same cycle. This is where supplements and vitamins come in.

When it comes to vitamins and supplements, be sure you invest in high-quality, medical grade options. There are companies that do third party testing to ensure quality. Unfortunately, reports from those companies reveal that with many vitamins and supplements, there's nothing but filler used. Don't waste your money. Do a little research so you know you're getting a high-quality supplement.

Our body can also signal our need for supplements. Take hair loss, for example. Hair loss can stem from a myriad of reasons, such as high stress, hormone changes, and thyroid issues. It can also come from too low or too high vitamin A, or low B vitamins.

Here are some of the vitamins I review the most with my clients. Instead of making a general recommendation for everyone to follow,

I typically work with my clients on a one-on-one basis for what their supplement needs are. Work with your naturopathic doctor to decide which ones would be right for you.

Probiotic

With probiotics, you're sending in the good guys to get rid of the bad bacteria in your gut. That way, you can absorb more nutrients from your food. It's amazing how our gut bacteria can impact our health in a positive or negative way. Disordered gut bacteria can impact our mental health, skin, and may even exacerbate depression or anxiety. The wrong gut bacteria can make it harder to lose weight.

Having the right gut bacteria can help regulate bowel movements, they can prevent or treat diarrhea, may help with weight loss, and evidence supports the role of probiotics in improving our immune systems[74].

I'd recommend taking a high-quality probiotic daily. Sauerkraut, kombucha, fermented vegetables, kimchi, kefir, yogurt, and sourdough bread are some probiotic food sources. If you think you're getting the stomach flu or not feeling well, take a probiotic and extra vitamin D to help it pass or not happen.

Magnesium

As a society, we're almost 80% deficient for magnesium! Low magnesium manifests itself in issues like anxiety, overthinking, and difficulty sleeping. When we have enough magnesium in our body, it creates a really calm environment, particularly at night. It can also help with general anxiety, leg cramps, and constipation.

Vitamin D3 to Help Heal Depression

Although multifaceted, depression (particularly in people who complain of having a lower mood in general), can be assisted by something as simple as vitamin D3. Seasonal depression usually happens in the winter, when we aren't in the sun, or the sun is far away. This type of depression can be particularly responsive to supplementation.

Whenever I hear that one of my clients is struggling with low mood, apathy, or clinical depression, I always recommend a vitamin D3 supplement right away. If your doctor will cooperate, drawing a vitamin D level is always good to have.

Some of my clients, within a day of starting vitamin D3 supplements, report feeling a difference. The correlation between vitamin D3 and our mood is sometimes astonishing. When it comes to depression, there's usually not just one thing causing it, however. You may need to see a doctor and get blood work done. Most doctors want to put you on medication right away, but there are more natural routes you can take first to see if they make a difference.

For example, high gut bacteria can cause depression symptoms. Working out helps elevate our mood and releases endorphins. A lot of small changes (working out, taking supplementation, getting in the sun more, doing mindset work with a counselor) can often make a difference—even though it doesn't work for everyone and medication can help.

Looking at any issues on blood work and vitamin deficiencies when dealing with depression and anxiety is helpful, even if it's not curative all the time. There are so many underlying issues that need to be examined before throwing medication at the problem. Nutrient deficiency is a prime example.

If you struggle with anxiety and depression, and medication isn't working very well, let's deal with any nutrient deficiencies as well. This ensures you're feeling your best and addressing all issues. You can have more confidence in all your health-related decisions.

B-complex and B-12 Vitamins

I love the B vitamins because they give us energy from our food, and they help us with anti-aging. They're so good for many things like lowering cholesterol, protecting our skin from sun damage, boosting hair growth, and reducing wrinkles. B vitamins are great for stress, too. The B-9 vitamin actually helps iron do it's job!

Without it, you don't get benefits from iron, which impacts us all the way to our red blood cells. If you're low in iron, you may also be low in your B vitamins, which help that iron be absorbed.

There are eight B vitamins, but you don't need to worry about supplementing individually. I recommend taking a B-complex with a B-12 vitamin, especially if you don't eat a lot of red meat. I do not recommend taking folic acid (which is synthetic). Instead, opt for a methylated version of the B-9 vitamin folate that should come in your B-complex supplement.

Omega-3

Omega 3's can help fight depression, anxiety, improve eye health, promote brain health, and reduce ADHD symptoms or metabolic syndrome. They're protective of our heart health[75] and can benefit optimal brain health. Omega 3's have an anti-inflammatory[76] effect, which can lead to decreased joint pain and better weight loss results.

I recommend starting with 500mg - 1,000mg, with combined DHA and EPA. With fish oil, you want to be careful because they can be low quality and have high mercury, so stick with a trusted, medical-grade supplement source.

FAQ

Frequently Asked Questions

1. **Can I do a cheat meal?** The problem with a cheat meal is that it can trigger your cravings to start again, forcing you to white knuckle back through them to get it under control. If you're going to have a cheat meal, plan ahead, and exercise caution. Make sure it's a special occasion, and not a cheat meal created simply from cravings.

   I want you to tell yourself that you can have anything you want, but you choose not to because you're feeling good. You don't want to go back to your old ways because of a cheat meal.

   Of course, I believe in being real world. You can have a cheat meal or food or item, but just call it food. Don't label it as *good* or *bad* food. If you want it, plan for it. Enjoy it. Then go back to eating foods that make you feel your best.

2. **If I'm trying to lose weight, should I have a calorie deficit?** When you satisfy the body, you don't want to be in a deficit. Unfortunately, that is what a lot of diets do. They put the body in deficit for calories and nutrients. As a general strategy, I don't recommend this because there are other areas we can focus on

first. You can start small with these nourishing habits first. The last thing I would focus on is calories. If you've tried everything else first, then you can calculate how many calories you need a day, and cut back from there.

3. **What is ketosis?** Nutritional ketosis is when your body burns fat (or ketones) instead of sugar. The diet typically consists of high fat, moderate protein, and low carbs in the form of fibrous veggies. I recommend the keto diet for people who have tried everything else and cannot seem to shed weight. It helps control craving and hunger.

4. **Do you recommend doing a detox?** Detoxing gives the body a break and clean toxins out of the liver. You can help with the process by drinking more water and avoiding alcohol, sugar, and other chemicals. The liver gets clogged by consuming alcohol, pesticides, corn sugars, toxins, fructose, and other environmental toxins. All these can cause fatty liver. If you want to help the liver detox, consume less of the above, take in more water, and turn to green leafy veggies like arugula.

5. **Should I drink alkalized water?** Unfortunately, drinking artificially alkaline water may deplete vital minerals for unusual reasons. It may make the body think it is alkaline, so the body does not need to hold on to its alkaline reserve minerals as much, and it eliminates some of them, making you even more deficient.

6. **Do I recommend supplements?** Yes, but on a case-by-case basis. I recommend focusing supplementation on what your body needs or symptoms you have. Focus on one at a time so you can see how they make you feel. I always recommend a good,

medical-grade quality supplement that cannot be purchased in most stores. They're third party tested and work. You can also "pulse" your vitamins, which means you go on and off as needed.

7. **Do you recommend digestive enzymes?** Enzymes are protein molecules that are essential for digesting food. They aid in providing energy for the body to repair organs, tissues, and cells. Basically, digestive enzymes create energy for later use. Without these very important enzymes, we wouldn't exist! There are two different types:

    a. Enzymes secreted in the gastrointestinal (GI) tract. These enzymes break down food and enable nutrients to be used in a variety of bodily functions. They react within the cell to create energy production and detoxification.

    b. Enzymes found in plant and animal food. Most are in: avocados, pineapples, bananas, mangoes, etc. Sprouts are the best for enzymes, as well as unripe papaya and pineapple.

    You can also take a supplemental digestive enzymes, if you think you may have a proplem with digestion. If you're wondering if these would fit for you, give it a try and see if anything changes with your GI tract or bowl movements.

8. **Is hair loss a sign of something wrong with the way I'm eating?** In extreme cases, it could be. Your hair needs protein and iron to stay healthy, along with omega-3 fatty acids, zinc, and vitamin A. Very low-calorie diets are often lacking in sufficient

nutrients and can stunt hair growth or leave hair dull and limp. If the nutritional deficiency is big enough—like for someone with an eating disorder—hair can fall out.

9. **How can I have better skin?** Everything we do affects our skin, from not getting enough sleep or water, to consuming too much sugar and smoking. I recently visited a traditional weight loss clinic and most of the ladies had dull, gray skin that lacked elasticity. The nurse drank a diet soda filled with chemicals and a bar loaded with fake sugar and additives. Our body can only take so much. There are consequences to everything we do, and our skin bears that brunt of that. Stick with the nourishing habits, and your skin will benefit!

ACKNOWLEDGMENTS

This book is also dedicated to all my Nourish Nutrition and Health clients past, present, and future. Thank you for trusting me with so many personal stories and moments from your life. You are the reason that I wrote this book and want to give back to others. All your wins make me so proud, and I have been thrilled to be on this journey helping you getting to your healthiest body. Keep going and remember . . . one nourishing habit at a time!

Thank God for my girlfriends! Don't know how I would get through life without you. You encourage me to follow my dreams and push me toward going for it.

To my business coach Natalie Eckdahl. Thank you for supporting me and providing resources and a community through the BizChix, Inc. You have encouraged me on paths to take that helped my business thrive. I am so grateful for you.

For my writing coach Katie Cross. Thank you for your guidance, expertise, and unconditional support.

For the entire book team—thank you for all the work you did behind the scenes in putting my book together and making my dream become a reality.

Thank you to Lisa Briggs for letting me use your beautiful home for my book cover shoot.

Thank you to my amazing photographer Vincent Shakir for the cover photo. You are so talented and easy to work with. You made me feel like a supermodel.

To my super-talented and God-loving makeup and hair guru Jessica Shakir. Thank you for making me feel confident and bringing out my inner radiance.

To my biz bestie Jolynn Swafford, thank you for always holding me accountable and pushing me out of my comfort zone.

ABOUT THE AUTHOR

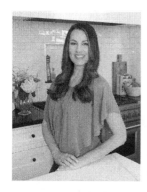 Julie Hefner is a certified, holistic nutritionist and health strategist who helps women get to their healthiest bodies.

She's the founder of Nourish Nutrition and Health in Newport Beach, California where she works with clients one-on-one or in groups, working both in person or virtually.

Julie believes that we must look at our health holistically, focusing on the root cause of what's not working in our body rather than just treating symptoms with a pill. She believes that through good quality foods, you can help heal almost everything in your body. Her goal is for you to feel balanced, energized, and empowered.

Julie invites you to join her on her crusade to health and wellness in both mind and body by connecting with her at www.nourishnutritionandhealth.com, on Instagram @nourish_nutrition, and Facebook at facebook.com/ nourishnutritionandhealth.

REFERENCES

1   Francesco, Cappuccio et al, "Sleep Duration and All-Cause Mortality: A Systematic Review and Meta-Analysis of Prospective Studies," SLEEP 33, no.5 (2010): 585-92.

2   Grandner, M; Sands-Lincoln, MR; Garland, Sheila; "Sleep Duration, Cardiovascular Disease and Proinflammatory Biomarkers." Nature and Science of Sleep, (2013), 5:93-107.

3   Hanlon, EC; Tasali, E; Leproult, R: Stuhr, KL; Donchek, E; deWit, H; Hillard, CJ; "Sleep Restriction Enhances the Daily Rhythm of Circulation Levels of Endocannabinoid 2-Arachidonoylglycerol." (March, 2016) SLEEP 1;39(3): 653-64.

4   Omar Mesarwi, MD; Jan Polak, Vsevolod Y. Polostsky. "Sleep Disorders and the Development of Insulin Resistance and Obesity." Endocrinol Metab Clin North Am. (2013). Sept; 42:3).

5   Spiegel, K; Tasali, E; Penev, P.; Van Cauter, E. "Bried Communication: Sleep Curltailment in Healthy Young Men is Associated with Decreased Leptin Levels, and Increased Hunger and Appetite." Ann Intern Med, (2004) Dec. 7; 141(11): 846-50.

6   Shahrad, Taheri; Ling Lin; Diane Austin; Terry Young; Emmanuel Mignot. "Short Sleep Duration Is Associated with Reduced Leptin, Elevated Ghrelin, and Increased Body Mass Index." PLOS Medicine (2004), 1(3); e62.

7   Luciana Besedovsky; Tanja Lange; Jan Born. "Sleep and Immune Function." European Journal of Physiology, (January 2012), 463(1): 121-137.

8   Janet M. Mullington; Norah S. Simpson; Hans K. Meier-Ewert; Monika Haack. "Sleep Loss and Inflammation." Best Practice & Research Clinical Endocrinology & Metabolism. (2010), 24(5): 775-784

9   R, Alina Masters Seithikurippu. "Melatonin, the Hormone of Darkness: From Sleep Promotion to Ebola Treatment." Brain Disorders & Therapy 04, no. 01 (February 19, 2015). Accessed August 14, 2019. doi:10.4172/2168-975x.1000151.

10   Reiter, Russel, Sergio Rosales-Corral, Dun-Xian Tan, Dario Acuna-Castroviejo, Lilan Qin, Shun-Fa Yang, and Kexin Xu. "Melatonin, a Full Service Anti-Cancer Agent: Inhibition of Initiation, Progression and Metastasis." International Journal of Molecular Sciences18, no. 4 (April 17, 2017): 843. Accessed August 14, 2019. doi:10.3390/ijms18040843.

11   Kawai, Nobuhiro, Noriaki Sakai, Masashi Okuro, Sachie Karakawa, Yosuke Tsuneyoshi, Noriko Kawasaki, Tomoko Takeda, Makoto Bannai, and Seiji Nishino. "The Sleep-Promoting and Hypothermic Effects of Glycine Are Mediated by NMDA Receptors in the Suprachiasmatic Nucleus." Neuropsychopharmacology 40, no. 6 (2014): 1405-416. Accessed August 13, 2019. doi:10.1038/npp.2014.326.

12   Hong, Ki-Bae, Yooheon Park, and Hyung Joo Suh. "Sleep-promoting Effects of a GABA/5-HTP Mixture: Behavioral Changes and Neuromodulation in an Invertebrate Model." Life Sciences 150 (February 26, 2016): 42-49. Accessed August 13, 2019. doi:10.1016/j.lfs.2016.02.086.

13   Harvard Health Publishing. "Keeping Kidney Stones at Bay." Harvard Health. April 2018. Accessed August 14, 2019. https://www.health.harvard.edu/kidney-disease-and-health/keeping-kidney-stones-at-bay.

14   Kato, Yoji, Tokio Domoto, Masanori Hiramitsu, Takao Katagiri, Kimiko Sato, Yukiko Miyake, Satomi Aoi, Katsuhide Ishihara, Hiromi Ikeda, Namiko Umei, Atsusi Takigawa, and Toshihide Harada. "Effect on Blood Pressure of Daily Lemon Ingestion and Walking." Journal of Nutrition and Metabolism (April 10, 2014): 1-6. Accessed August 13, 2019. doi:10.1155/2014/912684.

15   Mundell, E. J. "Are Americans Drinking Enough Water Every Day?" CBS News. April 26, 2016. Accessed August 14, 2019. https://www.cbsnews.com/news/are-americans-drinking-enough-water-every-day/.

16   Crutchfield, Stephen R., Cooper, Hellerstein, Daniel, and Joseph C. "The Benefits of Safer Drinking Water: The Value of Nitrate Reduction." SSRN. February 24, 2016. Accessed August 14, 2019. https://papers.ssrn.com/sol3/papers.cfm?abstract_id=2736657.

17   Fawell, John, and Mark J. Nieuwenhuijsen. "Contaminants in Drinking Water: Environmental Pollution and Health." British Medical Bulletin 68, no. 1 (December 2003): 199-208. Accessed August 17, 2019. doi:https://doi.org/10.1093/bmb/ldg027.

18   "Types of Drinking Water Contaminants." EPA. September 29, 2016. Accessed August 14, 2019. https://www.epa.gov/ccl/types-drinking-water-contaminants.

19   Nordqvist, Christian. "How Does Bisphenol A Affect Health?" Medical News Today. May 25, 2017. Accessed August 17, 2019. https://www.medicalnewstoday.com/articles/221205.php.

20   Patterson, Ruth E., and Dorothy D. Sears. "Metabolic Effects of Intermittent Fasting." Annual Review of Nutrition. July 17, 2017. Accessed August 14, 2019. https://www.annualreviews.org/doi/full/10.1146/annurev-nutr-071816-064634.

21   Klempel, Monica C., Cynthia M. Kroeger, Surabhi Bhutani, John F. Trepanowski, and Krista A. Varady. "Intermittent Fasting Combined with Calorie Restriction Is Effective for Weight Loss and Cardio-protection in Obese Women." Nutrition Journal 11, no. 1 (August 2006): 332-53. Accessed August 13, 2019. doi:10.1186/1475-2891-11-98.

22   Fasting as a Metabolic Stress Paradigm Selectively Amplifies Cortisol Secretory

Burst Mass and Delays the Time of Maximal Nyctohemeral Cortisol Concentrations in Healthy Men. The Journal of Clinical Endocrinology & Metabolism. (1996), 1 February, (81)2: 692-699.

23   Harris, Leanne, Sharon Hamilton, Liane B. Azevedo, Joan Olajide, Caroline De Brún, Gillian Waller, Vicki Whittaker, Tracey Sharp, Mike Lean, Catherine Hankey, and Louisa Ells. "Intermittent Fasting Interventions for Treatment of Overweight and Obesity in Adults." JBI Database of Systematic Reviews and Implementation Reports 16, no. 2 (February 2018): 507-47. Accessed August 10, 2019. doi:10.11124/jbisrir-2016-003248.

24   Martin, Bronwen, Mark P. Mattson, and Stuart Maudsley. "Caloric Restriction and Intermittent Fasting: Two Potential Diets for Successful Brain Aging." Ageing Research Reviews 5, no. 3 (August 2006): 332-53. Accessed August 13, 2019. doi:10.1016/j.arr.2006.04.002.

25   Mattson, M., and R. Wan. "Beneficial Effects of Intermittent Fasting and Caloric Restriction on the Cardiovascular and Cerebrovascular Systems." The Journal of Nutritional Biochemistry 16, no. 3 (March 2005): 129-37. Accessed August 13, 2019. doi:10.1016/j.jnutbio.2004.12.007.

26   Li, Liaoliao, Zhi Wang, and Zhiyi Zuo. "Chronic Intermittent Fasting Improves Cognitive Functions and Brain Structures in Mice." PLoS ONE 8, no. 6 (June 03, 2013). Accessed June 22, 2019. doi:10.1371/journal.pone.0066069.

27   Singh, Rumani, Dinesh Lakhanpal, Sushil Kumar, Sandeep Sharma, Hardeep Kataria, Manpreet Kaur, and Gurcharan Kaur. "Late-onset Intermittent Fasting Dietary Restriction as a Potential Intervention to Retard Age-associated Brain Function Impairments in Male Rats." Age 34, no. 4 (August 23, 2011): 917-33. Accessed June 22, 2019. doi:10.1007/s11357-011-9289-2.

28   Lettieri-Barbato, Daniele, Stefano Maria Cannata, Viviana Casagrande, Maria Rosa Ciriolo, and Katia Aquilano. "Time-controlled Fasting Prevents Aging-like Mitochondrial Changes Induced by Persistent Dietary Fat Overload in Skeletal Muscle." Plos One 13, no. 5 (2018). Accessed August 10, 2019. doi:10.1371/journal.pone.0195912.

29   Tillotson, James E. "We're Fat and Getting Fatter! What Is the Food Industry's Role?" Nutrition Today 37, no. 3 (March 28, 2014): 136-38. Accessed June 24, 2019. doi:10.1097/00017285-200205000-00014.

30   Roberts, Rosebud O., Lewis A. Roberts, Yonas E. Geda, Ruth H. Cha, V. Shane Pankratz, Helen M. Oconnor, David S. Knopman, and Ronald C. Petersen. "Relative Intake of Macronutrients Impacts Risk of Mild Cognitive Impairment or Dementia." Journal of Alzheimers Disease 32, no. 2 (June 12, 2012): 329-39. Accessed August 10, 2019. doi:10.3233/jad-2012-120862.

31   Chang, Chia-Yu, Der-Shin Ke, and Jen-Yin Chen. "Essential Fatty Acids and Human Brain." Acta Neurologica Taiwanica. December 2009. Accessed August 14, 2019. https://www.ncbi.nlm.nih.gov/pubmed/20329590.

32   Bredesen, Dale. The End of Alzheimer's: The First Program to Prevent and Reverse Cognitive Decline. 1st ed. Avery.

33   Skidmore College. "Diet helps shed pounds, release toxins and reduce oxidative stress." ScienceDaily. www.sciencedaily.com/releases/2017/01/170111184102.htm (accessed August 13, 2019).

34   Yue, Wei, Ji-Ping Wang, Yuebai Li, Ping Fan, Guijian Liu, Nan Zhang, Mark Conaway, Hongkun Wang, Kenneth S. Korach, Wayne Bocchinfuso, and Richard Santen. "Effects of Estrogen on Breast Cancer Development: Role of Estrogen Receptor Independent Mechanisms." International Journal of Cancer 127, no. 8 (March 2, 2016): 1748-757. Accessed August 11, 2019. doi:10.1002/ijc.25207.

35   "Polyunsaturated Fat." Www.heart.org. June 1, 2015. Accessed June 24, 2019. https://www.heart.org/en/healthy-living/healthy-eating/eat-smart/fats/polyunsaturated-fats.

36   St-Onge, Marie-Pierre, and Peter J. H. Jones. "Physiological Effects of Medium-Chain Triglycerides: Potential Agents in the Prevention of Obesity." The Journal of Nutrition 132, no. 3 (March 01, 2002): 329-32. Accessed August 11, 2019. doi:10.1093/jn/132.3.329.

37   "Office of Dietary Supplements - Omega-3 Fatty Acids." NIH Office of Dietary Supplements. July 9, 2019. Accessed August 14, 2019. https://ods.od.nih.gov/factsheets/Omega3FattyAcids-HealthProfessional/.

38   "Micronutrient Facts | Nutrition | CDC." Centers for Disease Control and Prevention. August 12, 2019. Accessed August 14, 2019. https://www.cdc.gov/nutrition/micronutrient-malnutrition/micronutrients/index.html.

39   Gunnars, Kris. "7 Proven Ways to Lose Weight on Autopilot (Without Counting Calories)." Healthline. May 11, 2018. Accessed June 22, 2019. https://www.healthline.com/nutrition/7-ways-to-lose-weight-without-counting-calories#section1.

40   Wang, Qiao-Ping, Yong Qi Lin, Lei Zhang, Yana A. Wilson, Lisa J. Oyston, James Cotterell, Yue Qi, Thang M. Khuong, Noman Bakhshi, Yoann Planchenault, Duncan T. Browman, Man Tat Lau, Tiffany A. Cole, Adam C.n. Wong, Stephen J. Simpson, Adam R. Cole, Josef M. Penninger, Herbert Herzog, and G. Gregory Neely. "Sucralose Promotes Food Intake through NPY and a Neuronal Fasting Response." Cell Metabolism 24, no. 1 (July 12, 2016): 75-90. Accessed August 11, 2019. doi:10.1016/j.cmet.2016.06.010.

41   Goodwin, Justin, Michael L. Neugent, Shin Yup Lee, Joshua H. Choe, Hyunsung Choi, Dana M. R. Jenkins, Robin J. Ruthenborg, Maddox W. Robinson, Ji Yun Jeong, Masaki Wake, Hajime Abe, Norihiko Takeda, Hiroko Endo, Masahiro Inoue, Zhenyu Xuan, Hyuntae Yoo, Min Chen, Jung-Mo Ahn, John D. Minna, Kristi L. Helke, Pankaj K. Singh, David B. Shackelford, and Jung-whan Kim. "The Distinct Metabolic Phenotype of Lung Squamous Cell Carcinoma Defines Selective Vulnerability to Glycolytic Inhibition." Nature News. May 26, 2017. Accessed August 14, 2019. https://www.nature.com/articles/ncomms15503.

42   "Added Sugar in the Diet." The Nutrition Source. January 02, 2019. Accessed August 14, 2019. https://www.hsph.harvard.edu/nutritionsource/carbohydrates/added-sugar-in-the-diet/.

43   "Know Your Limit for Added Sugars | Nutrition | CDC." Centers for Disease Control and Prevention. Accessed August 14, 2019. https://www.cdc.gov/nutrition/data-statistics/know-your-limit-for-added-sugars.html.

44   Wiss, David A., Nicole Avena, and Pedro Rada. "Sugar Addiction: From Evolution to Revolution." Frontiers in Psychiatry 9 (2018). Accessed August 11, 2019. doi:10.3389/fpsyt.2018.00545.

45   Crum, Alia J., William R. Corbin, Kelly D. Brownell, and Peter Salovey. "Mind over Milkshakes: Mindsets, Not Just Nutrients, Determine Ghrelin Response: Correction to Crum Et Al. (2011)." Health Psychology 30, no. 4 (July 2011): 429. Accessed August 14, 2019. doi:10.1037/a0024760.

46   News Center. "Stanford study links obesity to hormonal changes from lack sleep." News Center. December 6, 2004. Accessed August 14, 2019. https://med.stanford.edu/news/all-news/2004/stanford-study-links-obesity-to-hormonal-changes-from-lack-of-sleep.html.

47   Wurtman, Richard J., and Judith J. Wurtman. "Brain Serotonin, Carbohydrate-Craving, Obesity and Depression." Obesity Research 3, no. S4 (November 3, 1995): 477s-80s. Accessed June 25, 2019. doi:10.1002/j.1550-8528.1995.tb00215.x.

48   Benton, David, and Hayley A. Young. "Reducing Calorie Intake May Not Help You Lose Body Weight." Perspectives on Psychological Science 12, no. 5 (June 28, 2017): 703-14. Accessed June 10, 2019. doi:10.1177/1745691617690878.

49   Kirk, Erik P et al. "Minimal resistance training improves daily energy expenditure and fat oxidation." Medicine and science in sports and exercise vol. 41,5 (2009): 1122-9. doi:10.1249/MSS.0b013e318193c64e

50   Fredrickson, Barbara L. "The Role of Positive Emotions in Positive Psychology: The Broaden-and-build Theory of Positive Emotions." American Psychologist56, no. 3 (2001): 218-26. Accessed June 25, 2019. doi:10.1037//0003-066x.56.3.218.

51   Harbaugh, Casaundra N., and Michael W. Vasey. "When Do People Benefit from Gratitude Practice?" The Journal of Positive Psychology9, no. 6 (June 23, 2014): 535-46. Accessed June 25, 2019. doi:10.1080/17439760.2014.927905.

52   Korb, Alex, Ph.D. "Boosting Your Serotonin Activity." Psychology Today. November 17, 2011. Accessed August 14, 2019. https://www.psychologytoday.com/us/blog/prefrontal-nudity/201111/boosting-your-serotonin-activity.

53   Hatzigeorgiadis, Antonis, Nikos Zourbanos, Sofia Mpoumpaki, and Yannis Theodorakis. "Mechanisms Underlying the Self-talk–performance Relationship: The Effects of Motivational Self-talk on Self-confidence and Anxiety." Psychology of Sport and Exercise 10, no. 1 (January 2009): 186-92. Accessed June 28, 2019. doi:10.1016/j.psychsport.2008.07.009.

54   Amen, Daniel G. Change Your Brain, Change Your Life: Revised and Expanded

Edition. Place of Publication Not Identified: Piatkus Books, 2016.

55   Foster, Jane A., and Karen-Anne McVey Neufeld. "Gut-brain Axis: How the Microbiome Influences Anxiety and Depression." Trends in Neuroscience 36, no. 5 (May 2013): 305-12. Accessed June 28, 2019. doi:https://doi.org/10.1016/j.tins.2013.01.005.

56   Young, Simon N. "How to Increase Serotonin in the Human Brain without Drugs." J. Psychiatry Neuroscience 32, no. 6 (November 2007): 394-99. Accessed July 25, 2019. https://www.ncbi.nlm.nih.gov/pmc/articles/PMC2077351/.

57   Christiansen, Jens Juel, Christian B. Djurhuus, Claus H. Gravholt, Per Iversen, Jens Sandahl Christiansen, Ole Schmitz, Jørgen Weeke, Jens Otto Lunde Jørgensen, and Niels Møller. "Effects of Cortisol on Carbohydrate, Lipid, and Protein Metabolism: Studies of Acute Cortisol Withdrawal in Adrenocortical Failure." The Journal of Clinical Endocrinology & Metabolism 92, no. 9 (September 01, 2007): 3553-559. Accessed August 12, 2019. doi:10.1210/jc.2007-0445.

58   Trueb, Ralphm. "Oxidative Stress in Ageing of Hair." International Journal of Trichology 1, no. 1 (2009): 6-14. Accessed June 28, 2019. doi:10.4103/0974-7753.51923.

59   Shmerling, Robert H. "Why Does Hair Turn Gray?" Harvard Health Blog. August 14, 2017. Accessed August 14, 2019. https://www.health.harvard.edu/blog/hair-turn-gray-2017091812226.

60   Aschbacher, K., E. Epel, O.M. Wolkowitz, A.A. Prather, E. Puterman, and F.S. Dhabhar. "Maintenance of a Positive Outlook during Acute Stress Protects against Pro-inflammatory Reactivity and Future Depressive Symptoms." Brain, Behavior, and Immunity. November 18, 2011. Accessed August 17, 2019. https://www.sciencedirect.com/science/article/pii/S0889159111005708.

61   Gardner, Benjamin, Phillippa Lally, and Jane Wardle. "Making Health Habitual: The Psychology of 'habit-formation' and General Practice." British Journal of General Practice 62, no. 605 (2012): 664-66. Accessed June 10, 2019. doi:10.3399/bjgp12x659466.

62   Obradovich, Nick, Robyn Migliorini, Sara C. Mednick, and James H. Fowler. "Nighttime Temperature and Human Sleep Loss in a Changing Climate." Science Advances 3, no. 5 (2017). Accessed August 17, 2019. doi:10.1126/sciadv.1601555.

63   Halgamuge, M. N. "Pineal Melatonin Level Disruption in Humans Due to Electromagnetic Fields and ICNIRP Limits." Radiation Protection Dosimetry 154, no. 4 (2012): 405-16. Accessed August 17, 2019. doi:10.1093/rpd/ncs255.

64   Kahleova, Hana, Jan Irene Lloren, Andrew Mashchak, Martin Hill, and Gary E. Fraser. "Meal Frequency and Timing Are Associated with Changes in Body Mass Index in Adventist Health Study 2." The Journal of Nutrition, July 12, 2017, 1722-728. Accessed June 10, 2019. doi:10.3945/jn.116.244749.

65   Jeong, Ji Na. "Effect of Pre-meal Water Consumption on Energy Intake and Satiety in Non-obese Young Adults." Clinical Nutrition Research 7, no. 4 (October 2018): 291.

Accessed August 13, 2019. doi:10.7762/cnr.2018.7.4.291.

66   Spritzler, Franziska. "9 Proven Ways to Fix The Hormones That Control Your Weight." Healthline. March 07, 2016. Accessed August 17, 2019. https://www.healthline.com/nutrition/9-fixes-for-weight-hormones.

67   Pratt, Iain Stephen, Emma Jane Croager, and Michael Rosenberg. "The Mathematical Relationship between Dishware Size and Portion Size." Appetite 58, no. 1 (2012): 299-302. Accessed August 17, 2019. doi:10.1016/j.appet.2011.10.010.

68   "How to Use Fruits and Vegetables to Help Manage Your Weight | Healthy Weight | CDC." Centers for Disease Control and Prevention. November 9, 2015. Accessed August 17, 2019. https://www.cdc.gov/healthyweight/healthy_eating/fruits_vegetables.html.

69   "How to Use Fruits and Vegetables to Help Manage Your Weight | Healthy Weight | CDC." Centers for Disease Control and Prevention. Accessed August 17, 2019. https://www.cdc.gov/healthyweight/healthy_eating/fruits_vegetables.html.

70   Bonner, Michael Y., and Jack L. Arbiser. "The Antioxidant Paradox: What Are Antioxidants and How Should They Be Used in a Therapeutic Context for Cancer." Future Medicinal Chemistry 6, no. 12 (2014): 1413-422. Accessed August 17, 2019. doi:10.4155/fmc.14.86.

71   Laufer, E. M., T. J. Hartman, D. J. Baer, E. W. Gunter, J. F. Dorgan, W. S. Campbell, B. A. Clevidence, E. D. Brown, D. Albanes, J. T. Judd, and P. R. Taylor. "Effects of Moderate Alcohol Consumption on Folate and Vitamin B12 Status in Postmenopausal Women." European Journal of Clinical Nutrition 58, no. 11 (2004): 1518-524. Accessed August 17, 2019. doi:10.1038/sj.ejcn.1602002.

72   Abdulla, A., and B. Badawy. "A Review of the Effects of Alcohol on Carbohydrate Metabolism." Alcohol and Alcoholism, Autumn 1977, 120-36. Accessed August 13, 2019. doi:10.1093/oxfordjournals.alcalc.a044072.

73   Rubio-Tapia, Alberto, Robert A. Kyle, Edward L. Kaplan, Dwight R. Johnson, William Page, Frederick Erdtmann, Tricia L. Banter, W. Ray Kim, Tara K. Phelps, Brian D. Lahr, Alan R. Zinsmeister, L. Joseph Melton, III, and Joseph A. Murray. "Increased Prevalence and Mortality in Undiagnosed Celiac Disease." Yearbook of Medicine 2009 (July 2009): 88-93. Accessed August 14, 2019. doi:10.1016/s0084-3873(09)79541-0.

74   Khalesi, Saman, Nick Bellissimo, Corneel Vandelanotte, Susan Williams, Dragana Stanley, and Christopher Irwin. "A Review of Probiotic Supplementation in Healthy Adults: Helpful or Hype?" European Journal of Clinical Nutrition 73, no. 1 (January 26, 2018): 24–37. https://doi.org/10.1038/s41430-018-0135-9.

75   Harvard Health Publishing. "Should You Be Taking an Omega-3 Supplement?" Harvard Health, April 2019. https://www.health.harvard.edu/staying-healthy/should-you-be-taking-an-omega-3-supplement.

76   Swanson, Danielle, Robert Block, and Shaker A. Mousa. "Omega-3 Fatty Acids EPA and DHA: Health Benefits Throughout Life." Advances in Nutrition 3, no. 1 (January 2012): 1–7. https://doi.org/10.3945/an.111.000893.

Made in the USA
San Bernardino, CA
12 December 2019